Praise for *Living with Inattentive ADHD*

"In a world where ADHD is misrepresented by the media, social influencers, and the anti-psychiatry movement, it is refreshing to read Cynthia Hammer's candid and illuminating account of her struggles with inattentive ADHD and her path to recovery. Anyone who wants to know what it means to live with ADHD, needs to read this book."

> —Stephen V. Faraone, Ph.D., distinguished professor and Vice Chair for Research, Department of Psychiatry, Norton College of Medicine at SUNY Upstate Medical University

"With wisdom and humor in equal measure, Cynthia Hammer has written a highly readable and useful book on ADHD. She never spares the reader from the pain of this devastating disorder, and yet she offers a positive and optimistic view on how to live with ADHD. I highly recommend this book to lay and professional readers alike."

> —Rakesh Jain, MD, MPH, Associate Clinical Professor, Department of Psychiatry and Behavioral Sciences, University of Texas Medical School

"Cynthia Hammer has packed a lifetime of pain and joy into this page-turner of a memoir. She tells the poignant story of how she discovered later in life that she had ADHD and came to terms as best she could with all the damage it did (as well as the blessings it bestowed). This slim volume, written with precision and breath-taking honesty, is an inspiring tale, understated but as clear as the trumpets of Jericho."

> —Dr. Edward Hallowell, founder of Hallowell ADHD Centers

"Cynthia Hammer has spent decades immersed in the science and politics of ADHD, but her most powerful contribution is the bravery, humor, and skill that she has brought to illuminating her lifetime struggle with the disorder. Read this book for powerful insights into what it really feels like to live with this vexing, perplexing condition."

> —Katherine Ellison, author and Pulitzer Prize-winning journalist

"This book is wonderful. Cynthia's honesty, insight, and sense of humor about her lifelong ADHD will be both a comfort and inspiration to others."
—Kathleen G. Nadeau, Ph.D., Licensed Clinical Psychologist

"As a therapist, I often suggest books to my clients to help them understand their struggles and know they're not alone. Cynthia Hammer's *Living with Inattentive ADHD*, which describes her journey from grieving to healing, is such a book. You'll grieve alongside her as she discovers the truth about her diagnosis and the "new" reality of living with ADHD as an informed person. If you have ever questioned whether you have inattentive ADHD, *Living with Inattentive ADHD* will bring you clarity and a deep understanding of this topic. Cynthia's story shows that it's never too late to create a new path in life."
—Lisa Rabinowitz, LCPC, certified Gottman Therapist specializing
    in couples with ADHD

"Cynthia Hammer's brave memoir shows readers the ups and downs, the heart-breaks and thrills, of a life lived well, with purpose, *and* with ADHD."
—J. Russell Ramsay, Ph.D., ABPP, Professor of Clinical Psychology in
    Psychiatry, University of Pennsylvania Perelman School of Medicine

"Cynthia Hammer's *Living with Inattentive ADHD* is a compelling—and at times, harrowing—journey through a life lived with the disorder. Filled with valuable insights based on Cynthia's professional knowledge and personal experience, it is a tale of struggle, tragedy, growth, and, ultimately, hope."
—Brendan Mahan, M.Ed., M.S., host of ADHD Essentials podcast

"Cynthia Hammer has written one of the best personal accounts of the realities of adult ADHD. No matter where you are in your ADHD journey, you can learn much from her struggles—some of which are heart-wrenching—and her many insights and solutions. This memoir is indispensable for those who want to learn to live with ADHD."
—Alan P. Brown, ADHD/Productivity Coach

"Cynthia has turned a lifetime of challenging emotions and behaviors into a highly relatable memoir, in which those with ADHD will clearly recognize themselves. After reading her memoir, I no longer feel alone or ashamed of my missteps because from understanding comes growth."
—Caroline Stokes CEC, PCC, Executive Business Sustainability Coach

LIVING WITH INATTENTIVE ADHD

LIVING WITH INATTENTIVE ADHD

Climbing the Circular Staircase of Attention Deficit Hyperactivity Disorder

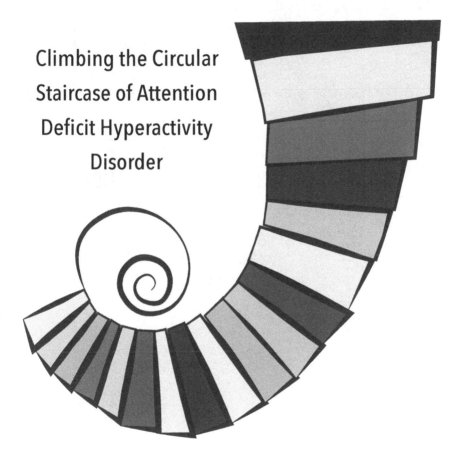

Cynthia Hammer, MSW

Foreword by William Dodson, MD

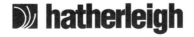

Hatherleigh Press is committed to preserving
and protecting the natural resources of the earth.
Environmentally responsible and sustainable practices
are embraced within the company's mission statement.

Visit us at www.hatherleighpress.com and register online
for free offers, discounts, special events, and more.

LIVING WITH INATTENTIVE ADHD

Library of Congress Cataloging-in-Publication Data is available.
ISBN: 978-1-57826-962-4

COVER AND INTERIOR DESIGN BY CAROLYN KASPER
COVER ART BY KRIS SYMER

Printed in the United States
10 9 8 7 6 5 4 3 2

I DEDICATE THIS BOOK to those who have sparked the neurodivergence movement, those speaking up for recognition and acceptance. Even as neurodivergent people learn new behaviors to better align with societal expectations, society, too, needs to learn to accommodate neurodivergence.

Contents

Foreword by Dr. William Dodson   *xiii*

Introduction: The Reality of ADHD   *xv*

Part One: A Bird's Eye View

Chapter One: I Could Only Shake My Head   3

Chapter Two: My Forgotten Childhood   15

Chapter Three: Early Risks and Challenges   21

Chapter Four: Conflicts with Mom   31

Part Two: Feeling Different, Damaged, and Overwhelmed

Chapter Five: A Mother's Sorrow   41

Chapter Six: The Night I Almost Died   49

Chapter Seven: ADHD in the Family   55

Chapter Eight: Raising Children with ADHD   63

Part Three: No Healing Without Understanding

Chapter Nine: Getting Answers   75

Chapter Ten: The Murky World of Diagnosis and Treatment   85

Chapter Eleven: Distraction and Inattention   97

Chapter Twelve: ADHD and Societal Niceties   111

Chapter Thirteen: Step-by-Step Improvements   121

Part Four: At Last, the Me I Was Meant to Be!

Chapter Fourteen: How Long Does It Take to Heal?   135

Chapter Fifteen: The Power of Positive Self-Talk   145

Chapter Sixteen: Finding the Humor in ADHD   151

Chapter Seventeen: Honoring My ADHD Positives   159

Chapter Eighteen: My ADHD Activism   167

Chapter Nineteen: Marriage and ADHD   181

Epilogue: Time is a Gift   187

Addendum: Symptoms of Inattentive ADHD with Examples for Adults 193

What Adults Need to Know Before and After an ADHD Diagnosis   199

Resources for Readers   209

About the Author   211

Note: The condition that I discuss in this book is called ADHD (Attention Deficit Hyperactivity Disorder) with three presentations:*

- Predominantly Inattentive (PI)

- Predominantly Hyperactive-Impulsive (H/I)

- Combined (C) where hyperactivity/impulsivity and inattention are present.

  * *Source: DSM-5*

I have ADHD-PI, but I prefer to say that I have inattentive ADHD.

Foreword by Dr. William Dodson

I HAVE NEVER MET A person with ADHD who was not constantly bedeviled by self-doubt in many forms:

- *I'm not the child my parents expected or wanted. I'm the outcast in the family.*

- *I'm constantly reminded that there's something wrong with me. I'm a fraud, an imposter.*

- *I'm unreliable. I can't do anything right. In fact, I rarely start projects, let alone finish them.*

- *I don't know how to raise my kids. I don't know how to protect them from my unreliability.*

- *I've always been so isolated and lonely.*

How could anyone survive living like this? The sad fact is that many people with ADHD don't and are lost to various addictions and even suicide.

No one can pull themselves out of such a pit without a very good guide who has been there. Cynthia Hammer is an expert one with her superb memoir, *Living with Inattentive ADHD*. She shows you, through personal example, how to live a rich and rewarding life despite the impediments and pitfalls of ADHD. She helps you learn from her journey, so you don't have to struggle alone.

Because Cynthia Hammer knows ADHD from "lived experience," she possesses an enormous amount of "street cred" in this candid, often harrowing book. She struggled with ADHD throughout her childhood, although the condition was not yet recognized. She continued to struggle as an adult and wasn't diagnosed until age 49.

Until then, she had to decipher the mysteries of her life without clues or guidance. Yet she was able to tame the self-doubt and shame that torment every person with ADHD. In 1992 she founded one of the first non-profits for adults with ADHD, and is currently the director of the non-profit Inattentive ADHD Coalition (www.iadhd.org), with a mission that children and adults with inattentive ADHD are diagnosed early and correctly.

The most important lesson you will take from this book is hope. Cynthia Hammer has done much more than talk and write about life with ADHD. She has walked the walk. The success she has achieved as a wife, mother, and activist shows that we, too, can make that journey. Cynthia's hard-earned "street cred" provides us with a rare gift that will help us live better lives.

I wish I had this precious resource available to me and to my patients through my many years diagnosing and treating ADHD.

William Dodson, M.D.
Board-Certified Psychiatrist Specializing in Adults with ADHD

INTRODUCTION

The Reality of ADHD

WHEN SOMEONE REMARKS IN an offhand way, "I think I have a bit of ADHD, too" or "Everyone is distracted at some point" or "Being forgetful is commonplace," their comments—regardless of whether or not they are aware of it—are hurtful to those of us who have ADHD. Friends and acquaintances believe they are compassionate when they tell us they share our experiences and that they relate to the difficulties we have in life. However, when someone jokes about, trivializes or even dismisses it altogether, they do not realize the harm they cause to someone with this perplexing, life-altering condition.

If you do not have ADHD, it is too easy to misunderstand or underestimate its seriousness. Many people believe it does not exist, that it is just a phony diagnosis promoted by the healthcare and pharmaceutical industries. The reality is far different, as I hope my story shows. Even those with mild ADHD (like me) struggle with shame and guilt when we do not understand why we act in certain ways. Until our diagnosis we do not have an explanation for why we say and do certain things or why we did not do or say the things we should have.

The effects of my ADHD were hard to explain to myself, let alone to my family and friends. How could anyone understand? Could they even relate to my calling a hotel in Boston to confirm a reservation I had made for my husband and me, only to be told by the hotel that they had no record of our reservation? I called the travel agency and they told me I had four online accounts, which was true. I opened a new one every time I forgot my password. When they eventually found my reservation, I had booked us for days we were not planning to be in Boston. All I could do was swallow my embarrassment, pay the $25 cancellation fee and hustle to locate another hotel.

That same week I left my purse in a supermarket and did not realize it was missing until they called me. That evening I planned to meet with Tacoma Wheelmen's Cycling Club members. We were going to Vancouver Island for a two-week trip and were meeting to review the final details. No one was there when I arrived at the meeting place with appetizers. I was at the right house but on the wrong night.

The following morning I was to attend a training seminar that began at 9 am. While driving there I glanced at the announcement and saw that the seminar started at 8:30 am. When I arrived late, I glanced at the announcement again and noticed that the event was scheduled for the previous Wednesday. I went to my office in a foul mood, determined to sort this out, and called the event organizers who told me the event was still on. Surprise! After all, I had the right date—their secretary had made a mistake in the announcement. Sometimes even neuro-normal people make mistakes!

I suppressed my annoyance and, in my sweetest voice said, "I am so relieved to learn that I haven't missed the meeting. Thank you so much."

I then madly drove back to the seminar. Maybe my dreadful week was turning a corner.

After reading these stories you may not believe that my ADHD is mild, yet you can see that it is bad enough. I say my ADHD is mild because I have no co-occurring conditions; I grew up in a home environment with expectations and structure which helped me to be moderately successful. About 25 percent of people with ADHD have no co-occurring conditions, while 50 percent or more have depression and/ or anxiety in addition to their ADHD—particularly if their diagnosis is delayed.

I wasn't diagnosed and treated for ADHD until I was 49. I graduated from college and graduate school, had a career in social work, was married, and the mother of three sons. There were areas of my life where I performed poorly but believed that was just my "personality." It never occurred to me that anything was unusual about how my brain worked until I received my diagnosis.

In writing this book I want to provide readers with an understanding of what ADHD is and how it affects a person's life. I want you, my reader, to develop empathy for those with ADHD who struggle to fit in, rarely believing they do or will. I want parents concerned about their children to learn that life with ADHD can provide many joys and satisfactions. Most of all I want people with ADHD to realize they are not alone, that they should not feel stigmatized by their condition and that there are ways to not only cope but to thrive and be content.

Like some people with ADHD, I was sad when officially told I had this disorder. I was ashamed that there was "something wrong with me" and bewildered that I had not known years earlier. I grieved about the difficulties and losses I suffered because of my undiagnosed condition.

It took years to accept myself as a valuable person who, incidentally, has inattentive ADHD. After accepting my diagnosis and understanding how it affected my behavior, I worked hard to reduce its negative impact. What helped was to tell myself repeatedly, "Getting a diagnosis for inattentive ADHD changes nothing. Everything in your life is the same. Nothing is worse, except now you have a name for it and are getting help. Being diagnosed and treated for my inattentive ADHD improves my life; hiding from it or denying it exists does not help."

Medication made an enormous difference in how I performed. Once I started on medication, countless issues that had challenged me no longer did or at least not to the same degree. However, other improvements did not happen quickly. The medication immediately improved my life, but it took additional years to learn new behaviors and habits. It took years to build self-confidence and self-esteem based on the improved me.

Slowly I became happy that I had been diagnosed. My sadness and self-consciousness disappeared and, as my performance improved, I recognized the positives of having ADHD. While I will never be ADHD-free, I have made it an unimportant factor in my life and rarely think about having it.

I wrote this book with several goals in mind. First, to describe problems in my life that are ADHD-related, second, to explain the strategies and tactics I employed to improve my life and finally, to describe the positives of having ADHD. I want readers to understand that while there are challenges with this disorder, there is more to life than "having a disorder."

As I describe my minor problems you might say, "Well, I have done that, too!" or, "That sounds like me." All the behaviors associated with an ADHD diagnosis are behaviors that others have. What distinguishes someone with ADHD is the frequency and degree of those behaviors and their impact on a person's life. These behaviors exist on a continuum from rare and infrequent to often or even daily. Unfortunately, many people do not realize they have ADHD and few clinicians automatically screen for it in their patients.

When I give talks on ADHD I want to shed light on how serious the disorder can be. I explain, in general terms, that the desirable things in life—graduating from college, having steady employment, earning an adequate income and having an enduring and committed marriage—are less likely to be achieved by those with undiagnosed ADHD. The negative things in life—poor educational achievement, spotty employment, poor physical health, low income, alcoholism and other addictions, criminal records and marital infidelity and divorce—are more likely.

Medication would have helped me greatly years ago. Both medication and structure are instrumental in living a full and satisfying life with ADHD. When we are young, hopefully, our parents provide the structure we need; but as we get older, we need to create and maintain the structure for ourselves or delegate this task to someone else. Maintaining structure and discipline as I sit at a chronically cluttered desk is a continuing challenge, but medication and creating routines and habits have helped enormously.

I cannot stress the importance of an early diagnosis enough. Unfortunately, the media and "knowledgeable" people say ADHD is over-diagnosed, even though many ADHD professionals believe this is not the case. Most ADHD clinicians believe under-diagnosing ADHD is more concerning than over-diagnosing it. We know that children with inattentive ADHD continue to be under-diagnosed. Adults with inattentive

ADHD are often misdiagnosed with depression or anxiety and do not get the help they need.

Children diagnosed with ADHD usually have one or both parents with ADHD as well. Because an increasing number of clinicians have knowledge of ADHD in children, more parents discover their ADHD after learning about their child's ADHD. The fact that adults have ADHD is not new, but it is newly recognized.

I hope this book makes clear what ADHD is and how profoundly it affects a person's physical, mental, and emotional well-being. I also hope it is a celebration of the resilience and fortitude of those with this disorder, and a testament to our power to take charge of our lives and succeed with this condition. ADHD is part of my life but it does not define my life. My message about ADHD is profoundly optimistic: In the face of significant challenges, we can live satisfying lives. I know this is true for you and your loved ones, whether you have ADHD or know someone who does. Join me on this journey of learning, discovery, and healing.

Cynthia Hammer, MSW
Tacoma, Washington
August 1, 2023

PART ONE

A Bird's Eye View

CHAPTER ONE

I Could Only Shake My Head

A POLICE OFFICER STOPPED ME one day as I drove home along the Schuster Parkway in Tacoma, Washington.

"Young lady," he began. (I was 53 at the time.) "Do you realize you were going 52 miles an hour in a 40 mile-an-hour zone?"

"No, officer, I wasn't aware of that."

"I need to see your driver's license and insurance for the van."

I found my driver's license in my wallet, thankful it was where it should be, but I could not find the insurance in the Honda Odyssey's glove compartment.

"I'm giving you a warning for driving over the speed limit, but this is a ticket for driving without insurance. If you appear in court with proof of insurance, your $150 fine will be reduced."

I got the ticket on November 10. On November 21 my husband and I bought a Toyota Prius, and on November 30 I drove the Prius to my court appearance. The judge asked me for proof of insurance. I walked out to the Prius, retrieved the proof of insurance, and handed it to the clerk who gave it to the judge. The judge studied the proof of insurance and then reviewed the information about my ticket.

"Please step forward."

I promptly complied with his request.

"This insurance policy began on November 22 but your ticket is dated November 10."

There was a pause while he waited for me to explain, but I remained silent. I could not explain the discrepancy in dates.

Then the judge said, in astonishment, "This ticket is for a Honda Odyssey and this insurance is for a Toyota Prius."

I had shown up in court on the right day but had forgotten why I needed to be there. I was embarrassed at making such a foolish mistake but it was far from the first time.

"Clerk, please reschedule Mrs. Hammer for a future court date when she will appear before me with the Honda Odyssey's proof of insurance."

I returned to court on January 3 with the correct insurance certificate. I waited and waited, listening to the other court cases, but they never called me before the court was adjourned for the morning. Stunned, I pulled the notice from my pocket and saw that my court date was for the following week, January 10.

The clincher to my courtroom saga occurred when my husband Steve told me, "There are two glove compartments in the Odyssey. The proof of insurance is in the top one." When the police officer stopped me, I looked in the wrong glove compartment. The insurance was in the car all along. I could only shake my head. We had that Odyssey for eight years and I never realized it had two glove compartments!

If you occasionally do this sort of thing, you think nothing of it. However, when someone makes mistakes like this almost every day that is a different kettle of fish. Everyone is forgetful, distracted, and confused at one time or another, but when these patterns are embedded in your everyday life, you probably have ADHD.

Getting details wrong is common for people with this disorder. We initially get something wrong without realizing it, and once we have it wrong in our heads, we keep referring to the incorrect information, not realizing we got it wrong to start with.

People with ADHD are distractible. When we park the car we do not pay attention to where we parked it as we are already thinking about what we plan to buy in the store. We do not pay attention when someone mentions the title of the next book to read or when the book discussion group meets again. We half register what was said and blithely proceed with our half knowledge.

I have many examples of things I frequently do but still struggle to remember how to do them correctly.

On my drive to Seattle the road splits: if I turn right I head north to Seattle; if I turn left, I head south to Portland. Because both roads initially take me in the opposite direction from my intended destination. I get confused about which road to take. If I don't read the signs carefully, I often make the wrong choice.

In the front hall of our house there are two light switches. One turns on the front porch light, the other turns on the hall light. After 45 years in this house I still do not remember which switch is correct. To help me remember I tell myself, "The top switch is for the porch light." The next time I want to turn on the porch light I say, "The top switch is for . . ." but I can't remember what comes after that!

When entering Costco I show my membership card to the clerk and put it in my coat pocket so I can easily get it when checking out. Then at checkout I look for it in my wallet because that is where it's supposed to be. After not finding it there, I remember—it is in my pocket. I understand most people have memory problems, but with ADHD I forget where I put something that was in my hand only five minutes earlier.

Being diagnosed and treated for inattentive ADHD allowed me to develop tactics to deal with forgetfulness. I make lists. I mentally prepare for events so that in the moment I will not forget important information. I purposely pay attention when parking the car and sometimes take a photo of where I parked it. I have put labels on the front hall light switches so I know which one is which. I remind myself before I confront the right turn for Seattle that it will be a turn to the right. My brain gets confused but if I give it a moment, especially when it is not under pressure to perform, I make the correct choice.

However, these tactics don't erase the painful memories of my more seriously forgetful episodes.

Our son Charles attended a Montessori preschool held in the teacher's home. One day I dropped him off at the front gate, watched him walk to the door and drove off. Two hours later a neighbor who lived near the school called me. I forgot that preschool was closed that day, and Charles had been sitting on the steps for two hours, waiting for my return.

I was mortified. What did Charles think? What did the neighbor think?

When our son Jackson was 9, I drove him to his first day at a new school. The school was four miles away; he was to take the bus back home. I called the bus system when he did not appear by 4 pm. He had not gotten on the bus. I called the school principal; he did not know Jackson's whereabouts.

I was frantic. I called Steve and told him Jackson was missing. In desperation I drove to the school to search for him. By now, he had been missing for two hours. A half-mile from the school I saw him cheerfully walking home. When I honked he got in the car and I burst into tears. I was crying so hard I could not see where I was going and had to pull into a parking lot. A concerned woman driver pulled up to ask if I was all right.

"Everything is fine. My son who I thought was lost is found." I cried tears of joy that I found him, tears of relief that he was safe, but I embarrassed Jackson with my show of emotion.

"It's no big deal," he said. "It's nothing to cry about. You said you would pick me up after school. When you didn't show up, I went to the YMCA and then decided to walk home."

To him I had not shown up. No big deal. I didn't know if I told him to take the bus home or I would pick him up. Not able to count on my version, not able to count on my memory, I believed Jackson's version was the correct one.

When I cannot even remember the commitments I make to my sons, I have to wonder, "Do they think they can't count on their mother?" Years later when I shared my diagnosis with them, my sons—who knew the letters ADHD but did not realize the impact this disorder had on my life—said little. The New England way of dealing with issues is to suck it up and not complain. I was not forever saying, "There goes my darn ADHD again." And they never asked me, "Do you think your ADHD is why you forgot to pick me up so many years ago?" We simply did not talk about it.

Even my husband Steve still does not have a good understanding of my ADHD and its effects on my life. It is for this reason that I believe most people with ADHD try to keep their struggles private—no one understands. That is why going to a conference with 800 other adults who have this disorder is an immense relief and a joyous occasion. We have "permission" to be who we are.

Having ADHD is like having arthritis—a hidden disorder. Others are rarely aware of our disability. If they are aware of some bizarre things we do or say, they chalk it up to our being unusual, not to our having a disorder. It is the rare person without ADHD who recognizes it. However, people with ADHD seem to have special antennae that recognize it in others who remain unaware they have this disorder.

Since my diagnosis I see people all the time who don't know they are living, day in and day out, with ADHD. Why is that? The most conservative estimate is that 4.4% of the population has ADHD, meaning one adult in every 25 I meet has it, but fewer than 20 percent have been diagnosed.

Several years ago Steve, Charles and I went on vacation to a remote location in Montana. Steve made reservations at a bed-and-breakfast, and I got ADHD vibes when I called the owner, Sally, to confirm our arrival. I did not tell Steve my suspicions because I knew he would roll his eyes. I kept my mouth shut (surprise, surprise) except to say to him, "We have reservations" (meaning the save-the-date kind).

So, why did I get ADHD vibes about Sally? Well . . .

- She had no record of our reservation when I called to confirm.
- When Steve called her three weeks earlier, she said she would send us literature. It never arrived.
- When I asked how much to send for the deposit, she could not remember what she charged.
- When I asked the cost of breakfast, she said, "$10 each," and then corrected herself: "No, $5."

- I reiterated the dates we would arrive, September 4, and depart, September 8. Immediately after my phone call with Sally, the fishing guide in Montana called me. Sally had called him and told him we were arriving on September 3!

After our arrival things were looking up. The bed-and-breakfast was well cared for—a spacious house with several rocking chairs on the front porch and a well-manicured lawn interspersed with flowerbeds of daisies and peonies. It was at the end of a long driveway with open grass fields in every direction under a blue sky that stretched from horizon to horizon.

Unfortunately, when I met Sally, the ADHD vibes also stretched from horizon to horizon. She had the frazzled, thrown-together appearance of many people with ADHD. She sat down to chat at our first morning's breakfast, lost track of time and burned the English muffins. (A reminder of episodes in my kitchen at home.)

The following day Sally, who said our breakfast would be at 8 am (to give the men a chance to eat before leaving to fish at 9 am), did not appear until 8:30 am. I had planned to bicycle for the day, but the key Sally gave me did not open the door to our room when I returned to get my sunglasses. Sally's husband was positive I inserted the key the wrong way. After a few tries he realized that Sally had given me the wrong key.

Perhaps I notice more people with ADHD because the numbers are increasing. One theory is that in a mobile society ADHD is more likely to increase because people with the condition are more likely to find one another. In a less mobile society someone with this disorder, having fewer choices, is unlikely to find a spouse with ADHD. This is significant because two people with ADHD are more likely to have children with the disorder, which strengthens the gene pool. People with ADHD naturally are attracted to one another—our patterns and rhythms synchronize.

If he spends long hours on the internet, it does not matter because she is out running a marathon. If she forgets to do the laundry, that is okay because he failed to buy the detergent. ADHD couples can happily coexist through many years of marriage. They find activities to do together or individually. Cycling and hiking are enjoyable to people with ADHD, as they require little structure, few rules, minimal organization and no planning. We enjoy activities where there is no need to reserve court time or find a partner.

Likewise, square dancing and contra dancing attract people with ADHD because little memory is needed. The caller tells the dancers what to do next. The music, the movement, the casual dress, and the relaxed atmosphere are tonics for those with ADHD. I believe Toastmasters attracts a disproportionate number of people with ADHD. We want to learn to communicate appropriately and may even want to learn to listen! When I gave a talk on being a "First Class Forgetter" at a Toastmaster's meeting, several people told me afterward it sounded like them. I nodded, saying to myself, "You probably have undiagnosed ADHD."

Recently, I joined a Great Books discussion group. Heated discussions on interesting ideas and topics attract people with this disorder. They like meaty conversations and find "chit-chat" a challenge and a waste of time. Once again I "recognized" the ADHDers among us because they could not "let go" when the discussion moved on. They had to have their say, even if their comments were no longer relevant.

If you are pining away for wild and crazy ADHD company, simply open your eyes and ears. You will find us. We are everywhere: Michael Phelps in the swimming pool, Simone Biles in the gymnasium, Adam

Levine in a rock band, Glenn Beck broadcasting the news, Lisa Lang writing the news, Richard Branson developing companies and Jamie Oliver cooking tasty dishes.

When I am open about having ADHD, I find I start unexpected conversations with people who say, "I have a son with ADHD," "My wife has ADHD," or "I sometimes wonder if I have ADHD." More so than with other mental disorders, the stigma for ADHD is profound and there is a widespread disbelief that a person has it or that it is a valid medical disorder. It is hard for people without ADHD to comprehend how globally ADHD affects a person's life.

Recently a woman with ADHD requested support from members of an online group. She wrote, "I am so tired of trying so hard. Despite trying, my partner still feels I am not trying hard enough. He does not recognize how difficult it is for me. I feel like I can't continue, that I can't go on living like this. Of course, I wouldn't do anything, but have any of you felt this way?"

Her comment made me wonder if I was fortunate to live for 49 years without knowing I had ADHD. What does learning you have ADHD do to a person's beliefs about herself? What impact does it have on a person who is no longer a child, yet not old enough to be secure in their self-image? How does a person who already has too many stresses in her life cope with the diagnosis? What if it's too much to handle, digest and accept? Perhaps her diagnosis comes with the expectation of improvement and the dismay is all the greater when improvement does not occur.

For some their diagnosis is a relief. They finally understand themselves and the reasons for their struggles but for others, the diagnosis is an additional burden, one more nail in the coffin of their presumed inadequacies. Their deficiencies become magnified in their minds, particularly when they learn about people who surmount their ADHD challenges while they still cannot get a grasp on their own. They go online to find others with ADHD who share their unhappiness to feel better temporarily. They think, "I am not alone. Others are flailing, the same as me."

I become sad and discouraged when I read posts like these. I know they don't share their shortcomings just to complain; they are asking for help, seeking ways forward. I know they want to create better lives for themselves, to be better partners, employees, parents, and friends but it all is too overwhelming. There are too many things to improve all at once.

I wrote this book to tell them about the path I took to improve, hoping they will improve as well.

I recommend patience. After I got my diagnosis I kept telling myself, "Nothing has changed. You only have a name for what has always been. A diagnosis for ADHD, unlike the diagnosis for some conditions, means you can get better."

But how do you get better? One step at a time. Your ADHD journey starts with one step, then another step, and another step after that. Over time your steps add up and you make significant progress.

Think of the simplest thing you can change to make the biggest difference. For some it may be getting to bed by 10 pm. For another it might be eating breakfast every morning. For me it was returning my credit card to its "home" in my wallet. Until my first step became a habit, I did not attempt a second step. But achieving my first good habit gave me the confidence to create a second good habit. I learned to talk encouragingly to myself. I took my baby steps and became more confident with each step.

Do not rush your ADHD journey. Take it one step at a time.

Myth: Everyone is a bit ADHD.

Fact: While everyone may have occasional typical ADHD behaviors, that does not mean they have ADHD. Just as many people are a few pounds overweight, that does not mean they are obese. Most people lose their keys, are late to class or a meeting, and have trouble delaying gratification occasionally, but these behaviors are not the same as having ADHD. With ADHD, the behaviors are frequent, and the reason is neurological. ADHD is a constant in the lives of people with this disorder. ADHD symptoms include inattention, weak impulse control, lack of focus, poor time management, procrastination, dysregulated emotions, and executive dysfunction.

CHAPTER TWO

My Forgotten Childhood

To BE DIAGNOSED WITH ADHD as an adult typically requires demonstrating that you had it as a child, and that you displayed symptoms before age 12. What a Catch-22! If you have ADHD you have a poor memory and can't remember instances that demonstrate having it as a child. Or the few instances you do remember that might be ADHD-related are not significant enough to persuade the diagnosing physician that you have the condition.

I am glad to learn that some knowledgeable diagnosticians are now saying it is inappropriate to expect adults with ADHD to remember incidents from their childhood. Today not remembering will not disqualify someone from obtaining a diagnosis as an adult. Fortunately I was diagnosed without stressing out about not having any or enough validating childhood memories.

As an adult I am not hyperactive, a hallmark of ADHD's more commonly diagnosed form. I get restless but don't have trouble "running or climbing at inappropriate times" or "trouble playing quietly" (as described in the DSM-V, the Diagnostic and Statistical Manual of Mental Disorders), yet maybe I did as a child. My parents are no longer alive to ask.

Although I have few childhood memories, let me tell you what I do remember. You can judge whether this was typical child/adolescent behavior or whether I acted this way because of undiagnosed ADHD.

I am the third child and the second girl in a family of two boys and two girls. I grew up in the factory town of Leominster, Massachusetts with a population of 20,000 located 50 miles west of Boston. Many parents of my classmates worked in one of the two plastic factories in town. We were one of the wealthier families and our home was a two-story, colonial-style house, dark gray with a fuchsia pink door. It was at the top of a hill on a street lined with maple trees, called Grove Avenue.

My father was proud to own this house. He occasionally sat in his car in front of it and asked of no one in particular, "Who lives in *this* beautiful home?" He earned his way through college and law school, and my mother, before marriage at age 25, was a secretary and lived with her parents. Owning this house was a dream come true for both of them.

In 1950 when I was seven years old, I spent a week at Children's Hospital in Boston for an evaluation. My parents must have had some concerns about me. I speculate it was my undiagnosed inattentive ADHD—not being aware of where my body was in space, my clumsiness and my lack of coordination. My parents often said I had the "heebie-jeebies," meaning the jitters. I knocked over my glass of milk at almost every meal. The doctors were unsure what was wrong, but they diagnosed me with probable Huntington's chorea or rheumatic fever.

Do the symptoms of Huntington's chorea replicate any symptoms of ADHD? From an internet search I learned that chorea, the most common involuntary movement problem in Huntington's disease, often leads to clumsiness. Physicians familiar with chorea describe the movements as "restlessness or fidgeting." Could the "restlessness or fidgeting" of chorea be the "squirming and fidgeting" symptoms of the Hyperactive-Impulsive type of ADHD? From my internet search I also learned that Huntington's chorea does not appear until adulthood. Maybe the doctors did not know that about Huntington's disease when they diagnosed me at age seven.

Some symptoms of rheumatic fever, my other diagnosis, are the same as ADHD—"jerky uncontrollable movements of the hands, feet, and face and a decrease in attention span." Like all medical professionals in 1950, the doctors who evaluated me did not know about ADHD. Since Huntington's chorea has no treatment, they might have diagnosed me with rheumatic fever because it has a treatment. I took penicillin, an antibiotic, for five years, which I am sure would go against good medical judgment today.

I never developed the other symptoms of rheumatic fever and never had problems with my heart, a common concern when a person has rheumatic fever. I occasionally returned to Children's Hospital for follow-up visits as I remember liking Dr. Barnes, who kept asking me to squeeze his hand with my right and left hand. (My sister remembers that I was kept home from school for a while but I don't remember this.)

My father's workbench was in the garage where my mother parked her beach wagon, commonly called a station wagon. The wooden workbench was about three feet high and five feet long and on one end there was a bank of drawers, also three feet tall. On top of the drawers my father stored several bottles of dangerous chemicals that he used in the vegetable garden or for chores around the house.

It was another long afternoon with only my four-year-old brother to play with, and we had run out of things to do. I had never climbed onto the workbench but I decided to try. It was a struggle for a 7-year-old, but I raised myself with my arms, swung one leg up, rolled forward, and got the rest of my body onto the workbench. I made it! I stood up and proudly exclaimed,

"Asa, look at me! I bet you can't climb up here!"

My brother stood watching me with wary but also curious and admiring eyes. He shook his head. He was not willing to try.

What was I going to do next? I didn't know myself but, having his attention, I turned and studied the bottles on top of the drawers. Asa continued to stare, sharing my fascination with these containers we were not supposed to touch. One was the size of a large soda bottle, partially filled with a clear liquid. I reached up, grabbed it and jumped down from the workbench.

"Here. This looks like water. Aren't you thirsty?"

I removed the cap and sniffed. The liquid had no smell and I held the bottle out to Asa.

"Take a sip."

He looked at me for reassurance.

"Here! Don't be a 'fraidy cat!'"

Years later, after my diagnosis, I wrote a short article for an ADHD publication, "Being Smart and Acting Stupid," describing the BSAS syndrome—acting without engaging my brain. Impulsivity, poor judgment and abnormal risk-taking are hallmarks of ADHD. People without this disorder sometimes act without engaging their brains but not to the degree, intensity or frequency of people with ADHD. My BSAS syndrome was certainly on display that day in our family garage.

Eager to please me, Asa took a swallow from the bottle I handed him and immediately burst into tears.

"My mouth burns! My stomach hurts! I want Mommy!"

"Please be quiet! Stop crying! You stay here!"

I rushed up the basement stairs and into the house. Without stopping to catch my breath, I yelled, "Mom, come quick! Asa drank something he shouldn't and he's feeling sick!"

She took him to the hospital where he had his stomach pumped. He returned home shortly, fully recovered. I don't remember the rest of the story but I probably got a spanking.

I didn't think jumping down an entire flight of stairs, all ten of them, would be considered ADHD behavior until I read the memoir of a woman with ADHD who mentions jumping a full flight of stairs as a child. So there are at least two of us who found this risk-taking activity a fun thing to do.

I was eight years old when I jumped stairs with my 10-year-old sister Melissa and my 12-year-old brother Elisha. They jumped from the eighth step to the landing below, farther than in previous jumping contests before they quit to do something else, but I persisted.

Could I jump more than they had?

Could I jump nine steps?

I safely did so!

How about ten steps, the entire flight?

I climbed to the top step and looked down. The distance was intimidating and I hesitated, but only momentarily. I could not suppress my impulsiveness and risk-taking. I wanted to surpass my siblings. I took a deep breath, crouched down and jumped with all my strength. I soared through space, but as I came in for the landing, my left ankle slammed into the newel post. I landed, spread-eagled, on the carpeted floor.

The pain in my ankle was excruciating. I cried out but no one heard me. Or maybe no one wanted to hear me. That is how it is with four rambunctious children in a family. It seemed like forever before my parents finished eating supper, and my father came out of the kitchen to find out why I was whimpering and pleading for help.

"Did you sprain your ankle?"

I didn't know the word's meaning but I said in my most pitiful voice, "Yes, I sprained it. See how swollen it is." He took a quick glance and drove me to the hospital for X-rays. I came home with a plaster cast on my ankle and lower left leg. Whether I jumped stairs ever again I don't recall. It hardly mattered. It certainly was not the last time I did something without thinking.

ADHD is a neurological disorder that affects the parts of the brain that help people plan, focus on, and execute tasks.

CHAPTER THREE

Early Risks and Challenges

A S I SAID BEFORE, MOST of my childhood is a total blank and my years in junior high are no exception. I only recall two of my teachers, Mr. Chase who taught history and Mrs. Cavanaugh who taught cooking, a required class for girls. I did not participate in clubs and do not remember any special friends except Kathy, who lived on the other side of town so we spent little time together.

Is ADHD the explanation for my poor memory? Or is this a common adolescent issue?

When I remember junior high, I think about loneliness. Because my birthday is in October I was younger than most of my classmates, but children with ADHD often appear and act younger than their peers. In junior high I wore braces and glasses and was flat-chested, so I was self-conscious and shy about my appearance.

The friends I had from grade school were dispersed into several other homerooms. We had different classes, different lunch periods and it was a much larger school. The one girlfriend I had in my neighborhood, Dale, became friends with Diane who shared her interest in boys. She no longer spent time with me. I was alone after school to entertain myself. I came home from school and got a glass of milk and a piece of mom's chocolate cake that I ate in the kitchen. Then I spent the rest of the afternoon lying on the carpet in the back of the living room, listening to the albums I received each month from the Columbia Record Club—*Sing-Along with Mitch Miller, My Fair Lady, South Pacific* and Elvis Presley. Despite my poor memory I listened to those albums so often that I still know many of the songs by heart.

Loneliness is certainly not unique to adolescents with ADHD but feeling like you don't fit in is common for children with this disorder. We are seen as (and often feel like) the square peg that struggles to fit into the round hole.

Another memory I have that might be ADHD-related is from a time when my parents were on vacation. I was 17, in my senior year of high school and was home with my older brother Elisha, now 21, on spring break from college and left in charge of Asa and me. My friend Paula came over for the afternoon. Paula was an outstanding athlete. She was of average height but had a sturdy body. Like me, she was an okay-but-not-great student but unlike me, she did not try to fit in. Paula went her own way but we had fun playing tennis and skiing together. I don't remember her dating or showing up at the weekly dances held each Saturday night in the large auditorium of the City Hall. Paula lived at home with her father; I never asked or found out about her mother.

I first met Paula when I took free tennis lessons at the courts in Leominster. These lessons were the only athletic outlet available for girls. When we started high school Paula was the friend I usually got into trouble with, so now I wonder if she had ADHD as well. Some of our pranks were climbing the school's rarely accessed backstairs to miss study hall and sunbathe on the roof, hanging a pair of men's underwear on the clothesline of our elderly English teacher, Miss Cooley, and sneaking out to Paula's car during school, which wasn't allowed, to listen to Alan Shepard's 1961 Space Flight. We were the obnoxious teenagers who wormed our way forward in the hour-long ski lift line at Mount Sunapee Ski Resort in New Hampshire, laughing at the angry stares or the irritated remarks we got.

This day I had new mischief in mind.

"Paula, my parents are out of town, and my brother is busy studying. How about going for a ride in my mother's beach wagon? We could go to the drive-in in Fitchburg and order root beer floats. My treat."

"That's a tempting offer . . . but wait, I thought you didn't have your license? You're always complaining about that."

"You know I don't but *you* have your driver's license and can give me whatever instruction I need. It isn't fair that my brother and sister got their licenses when they turned 16 and my parents won't let me. Come on! It'll be fun."

"You can count on me for anything fun but are you sure it will be all right? Are you sure we can go and come back without Elisha finding out and telling your parents? Aren't you in enough trouble with them already?"

"He's upstairs studying and will be at it for hours. Here are the car keys. No more talking. Let's go!"

We crept down the basement stairs, quietly opened the door to the garage and hesitated for only a moment.

I said, "Perhaps you should back the car out. It's a tight fit and I might hit the garage door frame."

"Okay, but that's all I'll do. This was your idea and I don't want to be responsible if anything goes wrong."

I loved my mother's beach wagon. It had three rows of seats, so when our family of six went anywhere, we always went in the beach wagon.

It had a white roof and hood and imitation brown wood panels along the sides. I loved its flared fins above the taillights and the recognizable Chevy grill that always looked like a wide, metallic smile to me.

After Paula backed the car out of the garage, I took over. I practiced on the infrequently traveled roads nearby learning to steer, step on the gas and apply the brakes. We doubled over with laughter as I alternated between flooring the gas and slamming on the brakes. Soon enough I felt ready to drive on Route 12, the main road to the two drive-ins that were eight miles away.

O ur choice of drive-ins was the Dairy Queen where we parked the car and went inside to order or the A&W Root Beer drive-in where we shouted our order into the microphone alongside the car. Carhops (girls our age in skimpy brown and tan outfits with matching hats) brought our food on trays that hooked onto the driver's side. We chose the A&W.

The hot dogs with mustard, relish and onions with a side of French fries were a real treat compared to the canned spaghetti I had been eating at home. But the root beer that came in thick, frost-covered glass mugs with the A&W logo on the side sticks in my memory. Never since have I had such great-tasting root beer!

So far, so good. We finished our food and were ready for the home stretch. However, when pulling out from the A&W I had to make a left-hand turn in front of oncoming traffic. This maneuver required driving skills that I did not possess. When I made the traffic stop to let me pull out and failed to signal that I was turning, a police officer appeared and asked for my driver's license.

Have I told you that I find it difficult, if not impossible, to lie? When he asked for my license I truthfully answered, "I don't have one."

The officer said, "You mean you don't have it with you?"

There was a pause while I pondered various possible answers but came up with nothing better than the truth again. "No," I said. "You heard me correctly, officer. I don't have a driver's license."

He was perplexed as he thought about what to do or say next.

"Well, I have to give you a ticket," he finally said, "and you will need to appear in court. And young lady, get out of the driver's seat right now. You are not allowed to drive."

My response was cheerful. "That's fine, officer. I don't mean to be troublesome. My friend Paula has her license and she can drive me home."

Once again my risk-taking tendencies had gotten me into trouble. When my parents returned from their enjoyable vacation (when you have to deliver unpleasant news timing is always important), I told them about my joy ride and the resulting ticket. I realize you are probably interested in what kind of punishment I received but I have to disappoint you—I don't remember that part of the story. However, living in a small community and having a father who is an attorney makes an enormous difference. My father went to the licensing bureau and got the ticket removed from my record.

Although I did not realize it at the time, I am quite sure, looking back that I was dealing with ADHD challenges in high school. The braces on my teeth had been removed but I still wore a retainer I took out whenever I ate. It embarrassed me to put it on my lunch tray so I always wrapped it in a napkin. After lunch I often threw the napkin in the trash.

Later in class I remembered, "My retainer!" and rushed to the cafeteria to dig through the garbage. If I found my retainer, I would be relieved. Some days I didn't find it and my parents had to buy me another.

Losing my retainers is one of the few "losing stories" I remember before my diagnosis. However, since losing things seems to go hand in hand with ADHD, I am sure I lost many items before I turned 49 and got my diagnosis. Today, all the additional expenses people incur because of their ADHD are humorously called "The ADHD Tax." Despite this, it is not funny how expensive ADHD can be. Until I wrote this book I never stopped to realize how expensive I had been—losing things, ruining or damaging items and incurring fines for late bill payments and overdrafts on the checking account.

Another challenge in high school was that the mechanics of writing were difficult for me. Children with ADHD often display deficits in tasks requiring coordination of complex movements such as handwriting.

In junior high most tests required us to fill in an answer or to choose the best of several options. In high school teachers expected us to write longer answers and compose essays as class assignments. What was a minor problem for me in my earlier schooling became an insurmountable one.

I am left-handed and my hand curves above my writing which causes my writing to be smudged. I didn't write legibly or fast. My hand tired quickly because I squeezed the pencil tightly and, as a result, had a permanent indentation on my middle finger.

Organizing my ideas was difficult. I remember struggling to write an essay about the Industrial Age for my high school history class. I sat at my mother's mahogany desk in my parents' bedroom with a pad of white paper with blue lines. I started, at least ten times, to write the essay and never got beyond the beginning sentences. I read over what I wrote, was displeased with it, bunched up each sheet of rejected writing and tossed it in the wastebasket, sighing and holding my head in my hands. I could not organize my ideas enough to produce a few tolerable sentences.

My father noticed my discouragement and came over to help. He quickly dictated a few opening sentences. "How could he do this so effortlessly?" I wondered. It must be because he was an attorney.

I hated writing—the mechanics and the thought processes—so I avoided it whenever possible, but I could not avoid it when taking the college entrance exams. These required a written essay. I sat dismayed, unable to think of what to write and how to start. I watched the students around me furiously filling page after page while I still had not begun. I completed only three messy pages before the proctor called, "Time's up. Put down your pencils. Close your booklets and pass them to the front of the room."

It was a blessing to learn in the 11th grade how to touch type. After that I typed my assignments, and writing got easier for me as I could type almost as fast as I thought.

After my diagnosis I learned that children with ADHD often have trouble with fine motor skills, jerky movements and poor hand control. This makes it hard for them to write quickly and legibly and explains why I gripped the pencil so tightly. Even after I took medication my handwriting challenges were not reduced.

Medication only helps about 80% of people with ADHD and alleviates only some of its symptoms. Which symptoms are reduced varies with the person. Although we have some symptoms in common, ADHD expresses itself differently with each person. It is an axiom of ADHD that if you have seen one person with ADHD, you have seen one person. All brains are as individual as fingerprints.

When I took a magnesium supplement at age 60, I was surprised that writing by hand became easier. The letters flowed and it was not as challenging to hold the pen. However, just like taking medication for

ADHD, I had to titrate the magnesium properly. If the dosage was too small, it did not make a difference. If it was too large, it might not work or cause undesirable side effects. The amount has to be within certain parameters to be effective. If I took 500 mg of magnesium every day and accumulated too much in my body, my hands got shaky. If I took too little, less than four times a week, my writing challenges returned.

I found, too, that writing with a pen about the width of a Sharpie relaxed my hand and improved my writing. It's hard to describe but, when holding a larger pen, my hand and mind seem to recognize where the pen is without gripping it so tightly. I still write slowly and prefer typing whenever that choice is available.

Of course, my writing difficulties are only one of the attendant burdens of ADHD, but still, improving any behavior is a victory that I need to celebrate.

Myth: ADHD is over-diagnosed.

Fact: There are many explanations for increased diagnostic rates, including:

- Improved awareness so more children and adults seek a diagnosis.
- A decreased stigma about neurodivergence makes parents and adults more willing to be diagnosed.
- The availability of many effective medications so more people are likely to seek a diagnosis
- More clinicians assess their patients/clients for ADHD, even when the patients/clients don't suspect they have this disorder.
- Research that shows a benefit to treating people with fewer than the prescribed number of symptoms

CHAPTER FOUR

Conflicts with Mom

I EXPECT ALL CHILDREN WITH ADHD try their parents' patience with their forgetfulness. We might mean well but we lose track of what they asked us to do. We appear obstinate when we find it hard to switch tasks when doing something we enjoy. "Clean up your room." "Put your things away." "Stop petting the dog when I'm talking to you!" "I told you an hour ago it was time for bed. Do I have to supervise your every move?"

Other times we cannot get ourselves to do what our parents want. We avoid tasks that sound boring or hard to perform. "Do I have to do that? Please give me something else to do." Or we start the task and get distracted by something along the way: "Okay. Today I'm going to surprise Mom. I'll clean up my room without her even asking. But what's this? The comic book I lost last week!" The next thing we know, we are engrossed in reading the comic book, completely forgetting the messy room and our vow to clean it up.

Kids with ADHD have trouble being punctual.

"How often have I told you we must leave by 8 am to get you to school on time? Do we have to have this argument every morning?"

"Mom, I'm ready."

"But you haven't combed your hair or put your homework in your backpack. Did you remember your lunch? I swear you'd wear out the patience of a saint."

Not only that, we are argumentative, frequently seeing only our side of a situation and we are reluctant to give up. We think of one reason after another for why our position is the right one.

The parent calls and says, "It's time for you to come home."

The child responds, "Why can't I stay longer? I'm having fun."

"It's almost suppertime."

"Last night we didn't eat until seven, 30 minutes from now. I can stay for 30 minutes and still get home in time for supper."

"Stop arguing with me. I want you home right now. It's your turn to set the table."

"What about this—I come home in 20 minutes? That leaves enough time to set the table."

"You wear me out! Why does it always have to be like this? You can stay but I say this against my better judgment. Part of me knows your 20 minutes will be longer than that. But I'm warning you—if you don't come home in time to set the table, you'll be grounded tomorrow."

I have two vivid memories of such interactions with my mother related to my ADHD traits of being stubborn and argumentative.

Once she bought me the latest style blouse from a store in Boston, a blue and white blouse with roll-up sleeves. Under different circumstances I would have liked the blouse but because my mother bought it for me,

I did not want it. I didn't try it on and handed it back to her, saying, "I don't like it. Why did you buy it for me? It looks stupid and I won't wear it." Not graciously accepting my mother's present was typical of my combative relationship with her. She took the blouse, abruptly turned and left the room without another word.

Another time, as a teenager, I talked back to my mother. I stood facing her in the front hall at the bottom of the stairs. I was 14 and at 5'7", we were the same height. I was overwrought and spoke aggressively, spitting the words out.

"Why are you always interfering in my life? I never get to do things the way I want! I hate living in this family."

"I have to do what I think is best," she replied wearily, worn down by our history. "Sometimes you do things or want to do things that aren't appropriate. Just because your older sister does something doesn't mean it's the right thing for you to do. It's no fun having a battle of words time and time again."

"That's what you always say." I shot back. "You never listen to me, to what I want. All I hear is, "You can't do this. You can't do that. I'm so sick of it! Why can't you be a better mother?"

The moment I spoke those words she slapped me hard on the left cheek. She had never done that! I pushed her too far. My eyes got wide and my jaw dropped. She stared at her upturned hand, stunned by what she had done. We stood there for a moment, not knowing what to do or say. I put my hand to my cheek and walked away with my head down and my shoulders slumped. I didn't want her to see I was crying.

After outgrowing adolescence I developed an affectionate relationship with my mother. Sometimes I went home for the weekend from college and occasionally brought a boyfriend. She waited for our arrival by the open front door, quickly engaged the new arrival in conversation and invited him into the kitchen for a "just out of the oven" treat.

After I married Steve and moved to Seattle I maintained close relations with my parents. I wrote, called, and had them join us on family vacations. My mother stayed with us for several weeks after the birth of each of my children. She said it was time to depart for home when I complained about how she did things. When worn out from childbirth I appreciated everything she did, but I wanted to do things my way as I got my strength back. If she moved the water glasses to a more convenient place in the cupboard, I asked why she moved them instead of acknowledging her brilliant decision. When I stopped being complimentary and appreciative, she left for home.

Perhaps my adventuresome spirit comes from my mother. She wanted my father to go with us on family trips but if he was unwilling to leave work, she took us without him. With four children, ages 12, 10, 8, and 5, she drove her station wagon from Fitchburg, Massachusetts to Harrisburg, Pennsylvania, an 800-mile round trip, to visit her family and my father's family. We children didn't have I-phones or tablets to keep us entertained during the endless drive, but we amused ourselves by keeping track of which state license plates we saw and playing the memory game of "I packed my bag and in it I put."

My father's mother still lived in the house where my father was born. Although it had electricity, gaslight fixtures remained in the hallways. Grandma Erb wore old ladies' clothes with black, lace-up, thick-heeled shoes. On one trip to Pennsylvania I got German measles and had to stay in a dark room and wear sunglasses until I recovered. Doctors at the time commonly believed that exposure to light when you had measles would make you lose your eyesight. Being confined to my room felt like the worst possible punishment.

My mother never attended college but she was comfortable talking with anyone. Every time she visited us in Washington state she arrived with tales from her seatmate on the plane that she talked with the entire flight. She was comfortable with herself and at ease with everyone. Even as a child I thought my mother was special. She was not exceptionally tall but when we shopped in crowded Filene's Bargain Basement and were separated, I could always locate her. To me, she always stood out.

I wanted to be an excellent student but was never in the top group. My report cards were usually all Bs (with the errant A in Physical Education).

I could not think of myself as intelligent because of all my stupid actions.

During high school I was put in a special study hall in the library with just one other student because we were the "troublemakers" in the regular study hall. The guidance counselor whose office adjoined the library supervised us although he was often elsewhere in the building. One day when he was out of his office, we snuck in and looked through his files. I found out my IQ was 135. Although I have little faith in IQ tests now, back then my IQ sustained me. Despite some of my unacceptable and foolish behaviors, I was smart!

In my senior year I applied to three colleges: the University of Massachusetts where I was confident of admission, Mount Holyoke, one of the highly selective "seven sisters" colleges, and Wheaton College, one of the seven less selective "little sisters" colleges. The admissions person at Mount Holyoke asked me why my score was 490 on my English SATs in my junior year and 650 in my senior year. She wondered if I was sick on the day with the lower score.

I had no explanation but variable performance without knowing why is a characteristic of ADHD. Perhaps I was less stressed the second time taking the test because I knew what to expect. I didn't understand then that my brain worked well in the right conditions and did not work well when I was stressed or distracted. I went to Wheaton, not Mount Holyoke, not realizing it was a poor choice for a person with ADHD who thrives on novelty and adventure.

Individuals with this disorder love stimulation and variety. It gets our adrenaline going and adrenaline wakes up our brains. Boredom is intolerable. Something boring never wakes up our brains. Being a student at Wheaton College in the village of Norton, Massachusetts was boring. The college of 800 women emptied on the weekends as they headed for various men's colleges, many as far away as a six-hour drive. That is how desperate we were to get away.

During the summer vacation after my first year of college, I worked as a server in an oceanfront hotel in New Jersey. Bob, a busboy from Colgate College, and I started dating so when I returned to Wheaton in the fall, I joined the women making the six-hour drive to Colgate. I also met my future husband, Steve, working at my summer job. He was a student at Brown University, only 45 minutes from Wheaton.

If I spent the weekend on campus I had few options for entertainment. I could study, play tennis or swim, and hang out in the "Smoker," a place on campus where students smoked, entertained visitors and played pool. I could also walk the half-mile to the local grocery store with a cafeteria counter.

How I recall the long, lonely weekends spent at Wheaton College. During my sophomore year I roomed by myself and had few friends. I learned the difference between being alone and being lonely. I never felt lonely if something engaged my mind.

After graduating from college with a major in economics I worked for a year in the trust department of a bank in Boston. I started dating Steve, who now was a 6-hour bus trip away in medical school in Montreal,

Canada. I hated the work in the bank but was afraid to leave, as it had been difficult for me to get a job. I was thankful when, a year later, I found a job teaching emotionally disturbed, blind children. This job persuaded me to become a social worker and I started my studies at the School of Social Work at Boston University. On March 1, 1969, during my first year as a student, Steve and I married. In June we moved to Seattle and I completed my second year of graduate school at the University of Washington. Since I received a government grant to work with the elderly, I trained as a geriatric social worker and continued my track record as an average student.

I worked for a few years before staying home to raise our three sons. I served as co-president of the Pierce County League of Women Voters during that time. When my youngest son started school I returned to work as a discharge planner three days a week at Tacoma General Hospital. Later still, I became a social worker at the Tobey Jones Retirement Community in Tacoma.

Shortly before graduating high school, I remember thinking, "I will do something remarkable with my life." After my diagnosis I read that most adults with ADHD have unrealistic self-images. We are doubly wounded when we are diagnosed—we have a disorder and realize we are not as special as we thought. We recall when we were sure we were right and everyone else was wrong. We remember when we were positive something was important and now realize it was not. After diagnosis and treatment we reflect on our earlier behaviors with insight and shame, recognizing how inappropriate we often were.

Long before my diagnosis I lost my belief that I was remarkable. I didn't know what caused my humbling experiences but they slowly undermined any lofty vision I had for my life. It would be many years before I rekindled my aspiration to do something meaningful with my life.

As of 2022, 2.5% of the world's population is about 200 million. An estimated 8.4% of children and 2.5% of adults in the world have ADHD.

https://www.psychiatry.org/patients-families/adhd/what-is-adhd

PART TWO

Feeling Different, Damaged, and Overwhelmed

CHAPTER FIVE

A Mother's Sorrow

AFTER I GRADUATED AS A social worker from the University of Washington, a senior center hired me as their activities director. Meanwhile, Steve, my husband, completed various surgical rotations. For his fourth year of training, he could do research in the University Hospital lab or join the Peace Corps and serve as a surgeon in Blantyre, Malawi.

I was eager to accompany him to Africa, even though we had a four-month-old daughter, Allison. She was born one month early, in August 1971, and was petite but healthy. Going to Africa with Steve as part of the Peace Corps appealed to my social work values. After graduating from college, I spent a summer in Nigeria with Operations Crossroads Africa and wanted to spend a year in another African country.

After our memorable year in Malawi, we returned to Seattle and settled in a small rental house in the city's south end. In Malawi our house had bars on the windows and solid exterior doors. The Europeans who lived in these homes before us feared being robbed. Back in the States where crime was more prevalent, our rental house had a rear door with a glass window that someone could easily break and picture windows without bars.

But the danger to Allison was inside, not outside, our house.

Steve and I took chloroquine, an anti-malaria pill, every week in Malawi. When we returned to Seattle we still needed to take the pills for two more weeks. I put four pills, two for each of us, in the pencil container on my desk in the den, perhaps thinking I would move them when I finished unpacking. Steve and I forgot to take the pills, and I forgot they were in the container on my desk.

Allison, now 17 months old, was inquisitive. One day she climbed onto the chair and then onto the desk, spilled the pencil container and swallowed the four green pills.

She stumbled, pale and glassy-eyed, out to where I sat in the living room. I did not know what could be the matter. In a panic I called her pediatrician. The receptionist asked, "Can I put you on hold?" the standard question when someone else was on the line, but my reply was not the usual one. With my heart hammering in my chest and my body shaking, I cried out, "No! I can't wait."

I hung up and ran out of the house to the busy street, Allison lying heavily in my arms, her eyes shut and her skin pale blue. I can't remember if I waved to a passing car or if a passing driver noticed my distress and stopped for us. He drove quickly to the Veterans Hospital, about a mile away, and pulled up to the front entrance. I ran inside with Allison in my arms. The hospital staff took her from me and rushed her into the emergency room.

A code blue sounded. Medical personnel rushed from all parts of the hospital to help, including Steve, who was a surgical resident there.

They got Allison breathing on a respirator, but she did not wake up. An ambulance took her to Children's Hospital where she died a few days later from a chloroquine overdose.

When Allison stumbled into the living room, I had no idea what was wrong. I only learned from the hospital that chloroquine was in her system and it was only then that I remembered where I had put the pills.

Why hadn't I put them in a safer place? I can only speculate.

Sometimes people with this ADHD do not know where to put something—we have not worked out how to organize our possessions so we impulsively put things down anywhere that seems to work as a temporary holding place. I might have been unpacking our suitcases, and when I came across the pills, I could not think of a better place to put them. With ADHD because of forgetfulness or being too busy, the temporary place becomes the permanent place.

As a physician Steve felt responsible that he had not remembered the pills and had not asked me where I had stored them. "I should have remembered," he said. "I should have asked you about them."

Steve was so grief-stricken that he talked of leaving the residency program. Yet he kept working at the hospital while I spent the days in the house crying. He recalls feeling detached from his work, unable to bring energy to tasks he usually loved. Even five months after Allison's death, his supervisors noted his apathy and asked whether he would like to take a leave of absence from the residency program.

We felt we had failed as parents and clung to each other.

I was three months pregnant with our second child and did not want to give birth. I worried if I could ever love another child. Could I keep another child safe?

I read in the newspaper about a woman who left her child in a hot car and the child died. The police arrested the woman and charged her with a crime. I heard about another woman who left her child unattended in the bathtub when she went to answer the phone. Her child drowned and the mother was charged with negligence.

Why wasn't I charged with a crime? Did I have special protection because Steve was training to be a surgeon? I was guilty but going to prison would not bring back my daughter.

I spent weeks in front of the TV, distracted by watching the Nixon impeachment hearings. Steve worked long hours at the hospital, leaving me alone to cry. I could not stop crying, but at least crying tired me out so I could fall asleep.

Dr. Michael Rothenburg, a Children's Hospital staff psychiatrist, spent several sessions with us. When we told him we would never recover from her death, he said, "You have been wounded. There will always be a scar, but you will recover." When we told him that we could not go on, he helped us realize that we could and that going on was what we needed to do.

I didn't dream all my life, and when I was told that everyone dreams, I thought, "I must have dreams but not remember them."

After Allison died I had a dream, one I will never forget—I watched in horror as she fell down a well, and I could not save her. I woke shaking. Dr. Rothenberg helped me understand the dream was part of my grief process. Again, he persuaded us that the best way forward was to keep our lives on track.

A woman once told the Buddha about her troublesome life. He told her to take a journey and knock on every door she passed to see if she could find a single person who did not have troubles or sorrows in life. The woman traveled for many years and knocked on thousands of doors but never found a home free of sorrow. The Buddha's teaching made me realize that everyone has burdens to bear.

Until Allison's death I expected my life always to be wonderful. After her death I lost that expectation.

We only started to believe a year and several months after Allison's death that we could make a new life for ourselves. Steve started his last surgical rotation in a community clinic in eastern Washington. We were in a new place and it felt like a new beginning. Spring had arrived, with sunshine and warmth. I helped care for a neighbor's two young girls along with Charles, our nine-month-old son, and Steve's workdays were less stressful. We played tennis on the courts that adjoined our apartment and hiked on the nearby hills covered with yellow balsamroot. It was here, in Wenatchee, that we began to look forward to the next stage of our lives. We would be living in Fort Knox, Kentucky for two years while Steve fulfilled his military commitment.

While at Fort Knox I met a friend's mother whose child had died years earlier. She told me, "I could never have gotten through my child's death without my religion."

I said, "Whatever religious beliefs I once had vanished. I can't believe in a God who let my daughter die." I didn't miss Him and stayed away from church and religion for most of my life. Occasionally, when things were rough, I thought about God testing Job. Was he testing me because I didn't believe in Him? Whenever I had the desire to pray, a voice in my head said, "You don't believe in God, so don't pray," and I did not.

Many years later I found a Unitarian Universalist Congregation in Tacoma and became a member. The church is a spiritual community without religious dogma. There I was open about my ADHD and the struggles I had in my life, and the congregation accepted me. I wish I had found this church much earlier.

Only after my diagnosis did I understand what caused Allison's death. My ADHD symptoms—disorganization, impulsivity, procrastination, distraction, and forgetfulness—explain my failure to protect my daughter.

I thought back to those other women—the one who left her child in a hot car and the one who left her child in a bathtub. I realized that these are the tragic mistakes people with undiagnosed ADHD might make. I imagined both these women had undiagnosed ADHD and felt sorry for them.

Myth: People who medicate their ADHD seek the easy way out.

Fact: Untreated ADHD can lead to several adverse outcomes, while treatment with ADHD medications reduces*:

- Accidental injuries and bone fractures
- Motor vehicle crashes
- Traumatic brain injury
- Burn injuries
- Emergency room admissions
- Suicide
- Premature death
- Teenage pregnancy
- Criminality
- Depression
- Drug and alcohol abuse
- Cigarette smoking
- Educational underachievement
- Sexually transmitted infections

* https://www.adhdevidence.org/ics

CHAPTER SIX

The Night I Almost Died

L ONG BEFORE MY DIAGNOSIS, there were several warning signs, as I was impulsive and reckless. I even had a near-death experience in the late 1980s that I now believe was because of my undiagnosed inattentive ADHD. I still get a queasy stomach and teary-eyed when I think of it. It was an incident I rarely mentioned and have never written about until now.

I took up sailboarding and had the perfect location for this sport: Purdy Bay, which has a tolerable temperature and water as calm as a lake. It was a safe place to sailboard; the bay was small with the far shore less than a mile away. The drawback was that the bay was 17 miles from our house, so I could not tell if the wind was up without calling a restaurant near the bay to find out.

Doing water starts separates the beginner from the advanced sail-boarder. For water starts, the sail lies in the water on the upwind side of the board. I push the sail up, so it fills with wind, and I am pulled out of the water and onto the board at the same time. I wanted to do water starts because it requires less effort and I could sail in high winds.

One day when I did not want to drive the 17 miles to Purdy Bay. I asked Steve to come with me to a put-in spot on Commencement Bay, an immense body of water down the hill from our house. The bay is so big that it has no far shore and massive freighters ply its waters when coming to the port in Tacoma. The water is cold and that day I had not worn a wetsuit, only my bathing suit with a life vest.

There are many reasons sailboarding on Commencement Bay is a foolish idea but I failed to notice the blinking lights: "Caution. Danger Ahead." Not only is the bay huge and cold but I never saw sailboarders on it. The only logical reason for choosing it is that it was close to home. Steve did not sailboard so he was unaware of my limited skills and did not understand the challenges posed by the bay. After he helped me rig my sailboard he returned to the car to read and occasionally looked out for me.

As soon as I climbed on my board, the wind picked up and my sail proved too large for the wind conditions. A more experienced sailboarder would have recognized the mismatch. The boom, the piece of equipment that attaches to the mast and provides structural support for the sail, kept being pushed out of my hands by the strong winds and the sail kept falling into the water.

I fought against the wind to pull it up, but again and again, it fell back into the water, and when it did, I fell backward off the board. The water was freezing. I was 30 feet from shore but now there was an outgoing tide and an offshore breeze. When I tried to sail to shore the sail luffed and the sailboard went "into irons"—it stopped moving forward. The wind and tide pushed me farther and farther from shore. I was exhausted and did not know what to do.

Then, without considering the consequences (which describes ADHD impulsivity to a "T"), I had the wrong-headed idea to take down the sail and paddle the board to shore but I still did not make headway. At this point, I should have called out to Steve. I should have abandoned the board and swum to shore but, in the moment, neither action occurred to me.

Maybe the thought of calling out seemed like an overreaction. Maybe I didn't want to abandon my sailboard or I didn't want to get into the cold water and swim. All I know is that after lowering the sail and being unsuccessful in paddling to shore, I had no idea what to do.

There was no way to get back to land as it was too far away. It was late in the day. There were few boats on the water and almost no one walking along the shore. The evening was coming on, the air was getting colder and I was in my wet bathing suit.

As the sailboard and I sped farther and farther from shore, I had to focus on staying balanced. I was amazed at my speed, at how quickly I left the shore miles behind. Brown's Point approached on my right, but I did not come near it. Vashon Island appeared on my left but I rushed right by. I was in the deep-water shipping channel, the waves surging higher and higher. I knew huge tankers took this channel at night to return to the Pacific Ocean.

With no boats on the water, I was alone and heading north.

I thought, "I am going to die tonight." Although terrified, I could not fall apart. *No negative thoughts, stay positive, stay focused, and be strong.*

I was moving as quickly as a kayaker shooting rapids in a raging river. If I were not afraid for my life I would have found it exciting, but I had to concentrate on staying balanced so I would not fall off the board. I heard a motorboat far behind me in the evening's stillness, but the sound faded.

The sun was setting and soon it would be dark. With nightfall I knew I would die. I told myself, *"If this is to be my last sunset I must enjoy it. I must focus only on the sunset."*

I did not know then that I had ADHD and that people with ADHD can hyperfocus. I did not know how satisfying and calming hyperfocusing feels to a scattered brain.

The sun was sinking and no one was coming to rescue me. I forced myself to stay calm, keep my mind clear and concentrate on the vivid colors of the sunset. In my mind I said goodbye to Steve and my children. I sat on my rushing board, keeping all thoughts out of my mind except for the setting sun. I still remember my peaceful feeling as I hyperfocused on the sunset.

Five minutes passed when I heard another motorboat coming in my direction. I was afraid to turn around and look, fearful I would fall off the board, become hypothermic in the cold water and die. But the sound of the motor continued to come closer and closer. Then a fireboat and its crew appeared beside me. They hauled me on board and one of them shouted into a phone, "We've got her!" I was shivering and unable to speak. They wrapped me in a blanket and gave me a hot drink. As we motored back to shore and the sky darkened, I was in shock and disbelief that I was safe and alive.

The first motorboat I heard that turned back was Steve in a friend's boat. They searched for me and turned back when they thought I could not have traveled fast enough to have gone any farther. They never imagined I was a great distance out on the bay. A man in a house overlooking Commencement Bay saw me in his telescope as the wind and waves rushed me northward. He saved my life by alerting the fireboat crew. He stayed on the phone and guided them as they searched for me because the high waves blocked me from their view.

The next day Steve and I went with a homemade apple pie to thank the firefighters. Then we thanked the man with the telescope although that would never be enough for saving my life.

I vowed to return to sailboarding but never did. Thirty-five years later, after abandoning my dream of doing water starts and sailing in high winds, I took up rowing as my new passion. It was only then that I returned to the waters of Commencement Bay, this time knowing I have ADHD and remembering I almost died because of it.

Adults with untreated ADHD die, on average, 12 years earlier than their peers without ADHD.

* https://www.additudemag.com/adhd-life-expectancy-russell-barkley

CHAPTER SEVEN

ADHD in the Family

I HAD AN EPIPHANY A few years before my diagnosis. As I walked into our basement and saw my half-finished project spread out in disarray on the workbench, something I started long before but lost interest in, I thought, for the first time, "This is something Bruce would do."

We did not realize Bruce, our middle son, had inattentive ADHD when he was in grade school but we knew from his behavior that he would likely flounder in a large middle school. We sent him to a private school where he was in a class of just twelve students. I don't remember what made me begin to connect inattentive ADHD with Bruce's challenges. Perhaps I first learned about the disorder at a presentation that started me thinking he might have it. I read the literature and shared what I read with Steve but the descriptions sometimes sounded like Bruce and other times not. They typically described the more common form of ADHD that included hyperactivity in addition to inattention and impulsivity. Bruce was not hyperactive.

Looking over the scattered traces of my forgotten project, I wondered if Steve had nagged me to pick it up and put it away as I nagged Bruce when he left things unfinished or did not pick up after himself. I wondered, for the first time, "Do I have inattentive ADHD like my son?"

After that I read more about inattentive ADHD but this time with myself, rather than Bruce, in mind. However, I found no literature about inattentive ADHD in adults. It was more confusing than helpful to read descriptions of inattentive ADHD in children. Certain behaviors fit me while others did not. I let any concern about having inattentive ADHD fade from my mind until that day in 1992 when my supervisor at work evaluated me in my office.

In two previous part-time jobs working as a hospital discharge planner and as a social worker on the staff of a multidisciplinary team assessing elderly patients, my supervisors had vague complaints about the lack of thoroughness in my work. They did not recognize that my challenges resulted from my undiagnosed and untreated disorder.

My younger brother Asa was diagnosed with ADHD as an adult, probably in the early 1980s when he was in his thirties. He took the bar examination to become an attorney several times before passing; maybe that was his impetus for being diagnosed. I had not seen him since 1969 when I moved to Seattle and did not know which of his behaviors got him diagnosed.

As a child, I knew my mother regularly took Asa to see a psychiatrist in Worcester, Massachusetts, 45 minutes away. At the time the primary tool psychiatrists had for helping people was talk therapy (my brother told me he played card games with the psychiatrist). I never knew why he saw a psychiatrist and he was not prescribed any medication. I don't remember any of my brother's behaviors that would have made me think two of my sons had the same issues. My only significant problem with my younger brother during my childhood was calling the neighbors and asking them to send Asa home because it was time for supper. He never came home without my phone call.

Today we understand that ADHD is highly inheritable but we did not know that in the 1980s, let alone in the 1950s. If one or two parents have ADHD, the likelihood that one or more children have it increases. A physician told me that second to a person's height, ADHD is the most inherited condition. Yet I had no reason to think my sons had ADHD just because my brother was diagnosed with this disorder.

It was not until the 1990s when interest in ADHD swelled and there was increased research into the causes that we began to develop a better understanding of how this disorder presents. Research by Stephen Faraone, Ph.D., shows that about 25% of children diagnosed with ADHD have a parent with the same disorder, and Ted Mandelkorn, MD, a pediatrician who exclusively diagnoses and treats children with ADHD, says, "Ninety percent of those with ADHD have a relative in the immediate or extended family with the disorder." Dr. Oren Mason once told me he had diagnosed ADHD in five generations of the same family.

Yet adults were (and still are) rarely diagnosed with ADHD. In the 1990s when I was diagnosed, researchers believed less than 20% of adults with ADHD were diagnosed. Although that percentage has increased with time, it is still too low. Population studies show that many adults with ADHD have never been diagnosed.

There are numerous reasons for this. Many adults are unaware they have ADHD, even when everyday tasks are burdensome. They may deny their difficulties, even when a friend points them out. Some adults were diagnosed as children and wrongly believe they outgrew it, or when they seek professional help, they are incorrectly diagnosed. According to Dr. William Dodson, an ADHD expert, clinicians frequently misdiagnose adults with ADHD as having a mood disorder. On average adults see

2.3 clinicians and complete 6.6 antidepressant trials before they are diagnosed correctly with attention deficit disorder.

Another reason adults are under-diagnosed is that many people and clinicians have a limited view of ADHD. They typically associate it with hyperactivity and poor focus. Adults often present without hyperactivity. If they were hyperactive as children, they learned to moderate their hyperactivity and express it in socially acceptable ways. They might doodle, jingle change in their pocket, wiggle a foot, tap a finger or walk about.

Adults with ADHD can have excellent focus and often can hyperfocus. The degree of our focus depends on our interest in the task. Sometimes parents refuse to accept a diagnosis of ADHD for their child, exclaiming, "How can you say he is inattentive when he spends hours playing video games?" When we hyperfocus, we lose track of time. When working on this memoir I sat at a computer in my home office, unaware of my surroundings. I was only aware of the writing on the computer screen. When I glanced away from the computer, I was surprised that it was dark outside and time to start dinner. Where did the hours go?

After reading a draft of this memoir, my sister Melissa suggested I include input from people who knew me before my diagnosis and treatment. What did they notice about me? Did they notice I was different from most adults?

So, I asked her, "Did you notice anything unusual about me growing up or when we took bike trips together?"

Her only response was, "I remember on one bike trip you told me how much Ritalin was helping you and then you told me you left it behind at the last motel." When I asked my oldest son he said, "I wasn't aware of you being unusual." When I asked my husband he said, "I knew you lacked caution and engaged in risky behaviors. You were thrill-seeking and sometimes you went too far. I knew this about you when we married but I just thought that was how you were."

He continued, "Remember when you went zip lining in Costa Rica? You were 67 years old and had no idea what you were getting into. I tried, without success, to prevent you from going. When you finished the course of ten different zip lines you told me how frightened you were but that it was impossible to turn back once you started the course. On one zip line you had to be rescued because you grasped the line too tightly. This made you stop in the middle where you dangled and twisted from side to side above the deepest canyon on the course. I tried to put checks on your risk-taking. Sometimes things worked out for you but other times you overestimated your abilities."

Unless our behaviors are way off the charts, it is unlikely anyone will think "brain disorder" when they encounter an adult with atypical behaviors. They will just label us "unusual," "irritating," "reckless," or "moody" or another disparaging term. Our inability to recognize mild and moderate brain disorders contributes to the small number of adults diagnosed with ADHD.

Although females are believed to have ADHD as often as males, the public image of ADHD is overwhelmingly of the hyperactive boy. For this reason girls—who more commonly have the inattentive type of ADHD—are diagnosed much less frequently than hyperactive boys are by a ratio of 1:3. It is theorized that those with the inattentive type of ADHD, which includes some boys, are underdiagnosed because they are daydreaming in class, not acting out and being disruptive.

Current knowledge about ADHD is that the disorder has three different presentations: Predominantly Hyperactive-Impulsive (about 10% of cases), Predominantly Inattentive (30% of cases) and Combined Presentation (about 60% of cases). During a person's life, the predominant presentation can vary. Undiagnosed ADHD, in any presentation, is damaging and needs an early diagnosis and treatment.

It was two additional years after we first thought that inattentive ADHD might explain Bruce's difficulties before we took him for an evaluation. We had different but still troublesome behaviors from our youngest son Jackson, but because he did well in school, it did not occur to us, until two years after Bruce's diagnosis, that he might have ADHD as well. Bruce's challenges involved not doing the things he should, while Jackson did things he should not.

I am sure that denial contributed to our delay in seeking help. No parent wants to believe there is something "wrong" with their children, something more concerning than typical, although annoying, behavior that warrants outside interventions and possibly medication. Until we accepted that our sons' "problem behaviors" were beyond our ability to rectify, I thought they were simply misbehaving, and if I disciplined them better, they would behave better.

ADHD is a disorder and a demoralizing label. My brother Asa had significant problems in life because of ADHD. He had trouble finishing high school and took years to graduate from a three-year business course at Babson College. He went on to study law but had trouble advancing in his career.

Often treatment for ADHD does not eliminate all the symptoms of the disorder. I never asked Asa if he continued to take medication when he worked as an attorney. Once they function better, it is not unusual for people mistakenly to believe, "I no longer need medication." When they stop taking it, their problem behaviors return and they are unaware of the change.

A friend called me about her son who graduated from college. He was hired for a wonderful job but was fired within a year. In talking with her, I learned that he stopped taking his ADHD medication when he graduated. He thought he only needed it to perform well in his studies, not appreciating medication's wide-ranging effects on all aspects of a person's performance. After he saw a psychiatrist in California who prescribed the needed medication, another company hired him and he became a valued employee.

What I knew about ADHD made me reluctant to associate my children with this disorder. Would I be consigning them to a bleak future? Wasn't it a handicapping condition? Once diagnosed that was it. Instead of focusing on how treatment brings improvement, I chose to deny the possibility that Bruce and Jackson had a disorder. It was more hopeful to believe that better parenting skills would make a difference than to think there was something that needed fixing.

Our oldest son, Charles, was no trouble. He was the model child. Why did the parenting methods I used to raise him not have the same result with my other sons? When we presented this conundrum to our family therapist, he said, "You aren't parenting your other sons the right way for them!" But what was the right way?

ADHD runs in families. Siblings of youth with ADHD and children of adults with ADHD are at high risk for ADHD and should be screened. About 25% of parents who have children with ADHD may require treatment for ADHD and/or co-occurring disorders.

CHAPTER EIGHT

Raising Children with ADHD

THANKFULLY CHARLES, OUR FIRSTBORN son, did not have ADHD. Dr. Amen says when parents of children with ADHD have a child without ADHD, they hold him up with great pride, proving they are good parents. Children with ADHD, especially when undiagnosed and untreated, often (and repeatedly) make their parents believe they are terrible parents, doing everything wrong in child-rearing. We were proud of our Charles, high-achieving and capable—and were equally bewildered, stymied and physically and emotionally drained by our other two sons.

Jackson, our youngest, had outstanding athletic ability but also an attitude and an impulsive mouth. Like our other sons, he played soccer—and if his coach said something Jackson did not like, he would say something back. His coach was a no-nonsense, I-am-the-boss kind of person. He dealt with Jackson by letting us know we were deficient parents for having an insolent child. He made sure we knew that if Jackson were his son such behavior would have been threatened or beaten out of him long ago. Word went up and down the line of parents about what our son said or did to provoke the coach. And so, even though our son was the star player on the team, going to his games brought us no pleasure as we tensely anticipated the coach's displeasure.

Although a good player when the ball came his way, Bruce usually had his mind on other things when the ball was elsewhere on the field. He would look at the grass or the clouds but never seemed to look at what was happening in the game. As the ball came up the field, his dad, the coach and other parents anxiously (and sometimes angrily) shouted at him, "Pay attention!" "Keep your mind on the game!" "The ball's coming your way!"

Moreover, of course, it was not only in recreation that my children proved a handful. Here are just a couple of my memories as an undiagnosed ADHD mother raising two sons with undiagnosed ADHD.

Problem One: No Space of My Own

When I worked at Tobey Jones Retirement Home, I listened to a presentation about the losses people experience when they move into a retirement home. The presenter asked each of us whether we had a space in our homes that was our special place, an area recognized as ours. A space no one violated or entered without permission. Staff members responded, naming a particular chair, the end of the living room sofa or a corner of a room that was their "special place."

I realized I had no special place. My sons with ADHD did not respect boundaries. I told them to stay out of my purse, out of my closet, out of my room, to not to use my possessions without asking, all to no avail. I knocked before entering their rooms, but they did not extend this courtesy to me.

My husband and I became resigned, albeit begrudgingly, to this state of affairs, although we periodically tried to work on it. For Charles, however, his brothers' misbehavior was very upsetting. Their violation of his space and possessions caused continual family upset. He got angry with us. "Why don't you do something about it?" he would demand. As I write this, I wonder, "Why *didn't* we do something? Why didn't we get him a key to his room?"

Our house is old and the original door key was lost, so it would have required taking the door latch to a locksmith, which was more complicated than I could manage. Being naive and idealistic, I didn't want to think one family member had to lock his room against two other family members. Foolishly, I believed more time and effort on my part would solve the problem that the younger boys would learn to respect the rights of others. How my thinking changed!

Bruce and Jackson said they would not care if someone took their stuff without asking, so they never believed that others might feel differently. They continually "assumed" the owner would not mind, even as I repeatedly told them, "I thought" and "I assumed" were unacceptable responses. They needed to ask. Of course, if the item they "borrowed" was lost or broken, that was that, unless someone, i.e., me, put in the time and energy to require the offending party to replace it and to make sure they did. As with the door latch, I could not provide consistency and follow-through.

Problem Two: Embarrassed and Shamed in Public

I still remember our first restaurant meal when we made a reasonable semblance of "a nice family out to dinner." Bruce and Jackson were 11 and 9 at the time, and while waiting for our meal, the waiter brought salsa and chips to our table. Both boys stayed seated, miracle upon miracle, and we talked, ate chips, and enjoyed one another's company. Usually Bruce and Jackson would fight with each other, both verbally and physically, while we waited for our food—and woe to the restaurant that took too long! We would remember and mark it as a place we would not return. The restaurant owners would probably be relieved to learn we had given them a black mark and would not be returning.

Usually, after ordering the food and awaiting its arrival, we would send Bruce and Jackson "out" to do . . . whatever they did. Then Steve, Charles and I sat and talked quietly while waiting for our food. When it arrived, one of us would look for the other boys and invite them back to the table. Invariably, they told tales of how they found a quarter by crawling under the cigarette machine, or how one of them had hit the other and that when hitting him back, they had accidentally hit another patron. They reported being bawled out or they had left the water running in the bathroom sink and it was now spilling onto the floor.

I know readers may have feelings about this, passing judgment on my husband and me as parents. Looking back on it now, I might pass a similar judgment, but at the time, we were worn out just from trying.

Attempting Discipline

Although I was spanked when I disobeyed as a child, my discipline method with my sons was to educate them about the right thing to do whenever they did something I disproved of. If it involved a punishment, I tried to fit the consequences to the misbehavior. Reminding them of desired behavior in advance sometimes led to the desired behavior, but it was an unending and exhausting process. Education, consequences, and reminders dominated my interactions with Bruce and Jackson.

"Bruce, where were you this afternoon? I checked to see if you had finished mowing the lawn and you were nowhere to be found. Now that you're here go out and finish the job."

"Jackson, we're going into the store now and I expect you to stay with me, not to pull things off the shelves and not wander away. Got it? Good."

"Jackson, you're not allowed into Charles' room without his permission. You need to put that Lego figure back."

"Bruce and Jackson, why are your coats on the kitchen counter? Pick them up and hang them in the closet. Wouldn't it be better to hang them up as soon as you came in the house?"

I said this day after day and then started tossing whatever they left on the kitchen counter down the basement stairs.

"Bruce and Jackson! Stop fighting right now! I can't drive safely! I'm going to pull over until you stop!"

I stopped the car and waited. When they quieted I started up again. I said nothing I was not ready to follow through on. I learned from behavior therapy that if you are inconsistent in your responses—if you sometimes ignore their fighting in the car and other times do not—it encourages the behavior. Stopping the car became an effective way to get the boys to cooperate.

However, it haunts me to remember one occasion when I stopped the car and said, "I parked in the handicapped parking space because I'm handicapped having you as my children!" I hope they don't remember I said that! It was an impulsive, ADHD thing to say.

A psychologist we saw for family therapy taught me behavior modification that used a point system, doling out rewards and punishments. Our sons earned positive or negative points daily. A certain number of negative points took away privileges while accumulating positive points earned things like watching a video, getting a pizza or going to the movies. If they wanted, they could save their points until they earned a bigger reward. I reviewed each child's behavior with him daily and recorded the points earned that day on the calendar. I tallied the weekly totals on Sundays. The system was helpful and the boys' behavior improved.

One month later, I was again in the therapist's office. He asked me how the point system was working. I didn't understand what he was asking me. I had forgotten the behavior program I had been using and had no explanation why. I returned home, determined to try again. My renewed effort faltered in two weeks. My untreated inattentive ADHD made it impossible for me to stick with a discipline system that required organization and consistency.

I tried another discipline method, *1-2-3-Magic*, developed by Thomas Phelan, Ph.D. I did not focus on all my sons' unacceptable behaviors, just the most trying ones. Each day when their behavior was unacceptable for the first time, I said, "That's a one." With the second occurrence, I said, "That's a two." When I started this system they exhausted me by testing my limits. I tried to be consistent. If I counted to three, they knew the consequences in advance and I imposed them immediately. After my sons learned I was serious, I rarely counted to three. However, as simple as *1-2-3-Magic* was, it was not simple enough for me.

Restrictions were difficult to enforce, especially when they argued. I was worn out trying to impose, monitor and remember what the restrictions were. I resorted to using *1-2-3 Magic* in a single situation—when the children insulted one another, especially at mealtime. The first offense led to a 25-cent deduction in allowance. A second offense and I took away another 25 cents. It worked and I stuck with it. It was effective and easier for me to enforce. Neither child wanted me to count higher than two and our evening meals became enjoyable. When you have children with ADHD, even small achievements are significant.

I could go on about our family travails but I think you get the picture. Those of you living in families with ADHD, know that you are not alone! Thankfully, in the midst of this turmoil, Bruce and Jackson were diagnosed and treated for ADHD—and a few years later so was I. That made a world of difference. As Bruce says, "People with ADHD (untreated) know what to do. They just can't get themselves to do it." And as Dr. Oren Mason says, "If there is ADHD in any family members, they all need treatment or too much stress remains." We are a treated family now. We have learned to do what we know we should.

Being a Parent with ADHD

After finally accepting the diagnosis for Bruce and Jackson, why did it take so long to recognize the disorder in me?

When I was diagnosed the descriptions of the symptoms lacked clarity and specificity and only described children. When I read the symptoms I said, "Yes, that describes me" for a few and "That doesn't sound like me" for others. There were nine symptoms of inattentive ADHD when I wondered if I had it. I only needed six of the symptoms but they also had to cause significant turmoil in my life.

In 1992, the symptoms I knew about were:

1. Missing details and becoming distracted easily. I had this symptom. Whenever I was engaged in one task, like making supper and thought of something else I needed to do, I went to do it and forgot whatever task I was doing previously.

2. Trouble focusing on the task at hand. I was not sure whether this symptom applied to me. If I needed to do something that I didn't want to do or did not interest me, I lost focus; but I could focus well and for long periods when the subject or activity was interesting.

3. Becoming bored quickly. I didn't know if I met the criteria. I got bored but did not believe it happened quickly. I avoided boring situations so, as an adult, boredom was rarely a problem.

4. Difficulty learning or organizing new information. I could learn things and loved to learn new and interesting things. I understood new information but my retention of new learning was poor. Yet I was a logical thinker and could explain things to others clearly, so I was unsure if this symptom applied to me.

5. Trouble completing homework or losing items needed to stay on task. If we replace "completing homework" with "completing housework," I agree. I had trouble. It was difficult for me to start and stay on task. Some of my brain thought someone else did the chores or I had already done them. It repeatedly surprised me to realize I was required to do the housework and that it would not be done if I did not do it. I acknowledged that I frequently lost items for projects I needed to complete.

6. Becoming confused easily or daydreaming frequently. I was not aware of becoming confused or daydreaming. Maybe the semantics confused me. I thought daydreaming was to engage in wishful thinking, not just thinking about things in my life. I researched "ADHD and daydreaming" and learned: "People with ADHD may hyperfocus while daydreaming. This is a more intense state than what people without ADHD experience when they are daydreaming. When people with ADHD daydream, you can call their name and they may not hear you. You may need to stand right in front of the person to get their attention." Had I known daydreaming presented this way, I would have checked this symptom. I remember being so engrossed in reading a book that I didn't hear my children calling my name until they waved their hands in front of the page I was reading.

7. Seeming not to listen when spoken to directly. I did this sometimes, but not always, so I questioned whether I qualified for this symptom.

8. Difficulty following instructions. This symptom was unclear to me. Did it mean I was unwilling to follow instructions or incapable of following them? I know I got better compliance from my sons if I broke tasks down sequentially, leading them through the process step-by-step. Perhaps it was the same with me—my brain got overwhelmed if anyone told me too many things to remember.

9. Processing information more slowly and with more mistakes than peers. I was unaware of processing information more slowly than others as I had no way of knowing how fast or slow others processed information. I knew how I did it but did not know I made mistakes others were unlikely to make. I typed the wrong dates with no awareness of doing so and left out keywords when writing, again with no awareness. I repeatedly called someone by the wrong name after it got stored in my brain incorrectly.

Based on these criteria I had only three symptoms—not enough to qualify for a diagnosis. Our knowledge and understanding of ADHD continue to evolve. See links in the Resource Section to the DSM-V description of this disorder and the World Health Organization's Adult ADHD Screening Test.

Myth: The common symptoms of ADHD include inattention, weak impulse control, lack of focus, poor time management, procrastination, dysregulated emotions and executive dysfunction.

Fact: ADHD is rooted in brain chemistry, not discipline. How do critics explain that the same parents challenged to raise their child with ADHD are often model parents for their children without ADHD?

PART THREE

No Healing Without Understanding

CHAPTER NINE

Getting Answers

A FTER THE TOBEY JONES Retirement Community hired me in 1987 as a geriatric social worker, I looked forward to working every day. My job provided variety and challenge, two qualities that appeal to a person with ADHD. Some days I gave tours to prospective residents; other days I would convince residents to accept personal assistance or participate in a physical therapy program. Another day I might guide a resident through the paperwork for end-of-life decisions.

The slow pace of speaking with elderly residents appealed to me. I relaxed in their company and enjoyed their life stories. The job required me to walk to three separate buildings, fulfilling my need for physical activity. I had independence, deciding what to do and when, other elements that appeal to someone with ADHD.

Yet my interactions with my teammates were not as smooth. Have you ever been in a situation where you believe co-workers don't like you, but you don't understand why? That is how it was for me with

Susan, the head nurse. I felt comfortable and at ease with the other nurses, but that may have been because they were more reluctant to show displeasure with me.

In the nursing home section of the retirement community, I had to chart every professional interaction I had with a patient. Slow, messy writing continued to plague me, as well as the challenge of organizing my thoughts and covering the necessary information in my chart notes. Sometimes that part of the job did not interest me, so I was not thorough or timely in my charting. If it ever occurred to me that some of my work problems could be ADHD-related, I pushed those thoughts to the back of my mind.

The previous administrator approved everything I did and never formally evaluated my work. After she left, Ann, the new administrator, planned to have annual evaluations of key staff members, but five years passed before she did so. Finally, Ann came to my office to evaluate me. My small and out-of-the-way office was perfect for a confidential meeting. Ann, a former nurse, was friendly, calm, and easy to talk with. She nestled on the cozy loveseat while I sat at my desk a few feet away.

"You're a mixed bag," she began. "I have difficulty evaluating your work because you do many tasks well but others poorly."

She pointed out areas where I needed to improve: being a team player, staying with a project until finished, and completing my most important tasks first.

"I can't understand why you tackle problems that aren't your responsibility," she went on. "The housekeepers told me you spent several hours rifling through Mrs. McAllister's personal papers after she died. That seemed an unusual thing for you to do."

My mind whirled, trying to think of a reasonable explanation, but there was not one.

"I don't know why I did that."

It was unusual behavior, inappropriate and unnecessary. Even now, after years of learning about this disorder, I cannot explain why I thought it urgently needed to be done and why I was the one to do it. I can't give a label to this behavior and never saw it described in the literature—doing something that seemed critical at the time and later realized it should not have been done at all.

Ann continued, "You had a wonderful idea to make a photographic display of the early life in this retirement community, but you didn't ask for permission before you spent time and money on it. You just jumped in without thinking who would hang the photos and where."

What could I say? She was pleasantly confronting me with my unacceptable behaviors. I sat there silent and mortified and struggled to maintain my composure.

Ann's grandson was diagnosed with ADHD so she was familiar with it. She knew my son Bruce was diagnosed three years before, in 1989 at age 13, and sometimes we shared information. Each of the behaviors that Ann described sounded like the behaviors of someone with ADHD.

After absorbing everything she said, I haltingly murmured, "I think I have Attention Deficit Disorder."

Ann's face lit up with a smile. "I think so, too." While Ann was pleased that she helped me identify my probable ADHD, my response differed.

I had trouble breathing and maintaining focus. My shoulders slumped, my stomach hollowed out, and my eyes watered. I have Attention Deficit Disorder. Something's the matter with me. I sat paralyzed as the meaning of these words sank in. It was 1992 and I was 49 years old. Why had I been clueless for so long?

Years later, when I realized how few adults ever learn about their undiagnosed ADHD, I was thankful that Ann had the knowledge and skill to encourage me to accept the possibility that I had

ADHD. Without her awareness I might never have gotten help and improved my life.

For three years, starting when he was 13, I went with Bruce for 15-minute monthly meetings with Dr. Smith, his pediatrician, a serious, middle-aged man. We sat in a drab conference room on child-sized chairs and reviewed Bruce's behavior from the preceding month.

"Bruce, how are things going in your life?"

"Pretty good, I guess. I'm on the basketball team at school, but every boy is on the team because so few boys are in our class. I've started playing tennis with my dad and I like that much better than basketball."

"How are you doing with your schoolwork?"

"We've started algebra and I can't say I like it. It's complicated. I seem to understand when Mom goes over the problems with me, but the next day in school I forget how to do it."

"Mom, do you have anything to report?"

"He seems happier. He co-operates in taking his medication and has better follow-through on his chores around the house. I haven't talked with his teachers to find out if they've noticed any differences. Did I tell you what finally got Steve to believe Bruce has inattentive ADHD? A teacher told us how in gym class Bruce would be off in space, absorbed, staring at the lights in the ceiling or gazing around the room, not fully taking part in the class."

After fifteen minutes of checking in and checking up, it was time to go. Bruce received a prescription for another month's supply of Ritalin— a controlled substance. We were required to get a new hand-written prescription every 30 days by law.

When we met next with Dr. Smith, after my evaluation by Ann, I said, "I think I have attention deficit disorder." Without hesitation, he responded, "You do."

He suspected but said nothing. This angered me, although I never revealed this to him. Years later, I read a question sent by a doctor to a newspaper advice columnist. He sat behind a woman at a concert and saw a blemish on her neck he thought was cancerous. He asked the columnist if he should have told her. The columnist said yes.

This made me think of Dr. Smith. If I had not told him I thought I had inattentive ADHD, would he ever have told me? Getting my diagnosis affected my life as much as it might for the woman with a cancerous growth. By not telling me his suspicions, Dr. Smith discounted the seriousness of my disability, which is neither fair nor ethical.

My friend Jane told me she had seen a therapist for over a year. When she figured out inattentive ADHD might cause her problems, she told her therapist. The therapist said, "I have thought so for a long time." Susan, understandably, was furious and asked, "Why didn't you tell me a long time ago?"

The therapist said, "I told someone once and it didn't go over well."

If a doctor suspects cancer, he does not avoid telling the patient because the patient might get upset. The therapist's reluctance to share her suspicions means the therapist did not realize how life-threatening it is to withhold that suspicion. Not life-threatening in that ADHD causes death, but life-threatening in diminishing one's potential, limiting all one wants to achieve and accomplish.

Dr. Smith observed me for fewer than 15 hours, yet he confidently diagnosed me. You may think this is strange, but once you know how ADHD presents itself, it's easy to recognize, especially if you spend more than an hour or two with someone. However, no physician today would make a diagnosis this way. We were still in the wild, wild west days of learning about ADHD. Now, a physician will do a thorough evaluation that will include checklists and reports, including input from significant others, because people with ADHD are notoriously poor self-observers.

I never asked Dr. Smith what made him determine I had ADHD, so I am only guessing based on typical behaviors. I interrupted when he talked with Bruce. I spoke of things that were irrelevant to the topic at hand. I went off track a lot, got restless, and expressed exasperation when the conversation was not interesting to me or repeated what we talked about in earlier meetings. I might have been late for appointments and been unaware of when the appointment was over. I probably had one more urgent thing to tell him even as he left the room to see his next patient.

When he made my diagnosis, I sat quietly with my hands on my lap, but my mind whirled with questions.

I reflected on my life. I have always felt different—and it was not a good feeling. However, since I did not know *how* or *why* I was different, I could not change myself to fit the mold. I was not a social misfit, as I had friends and participated in activities, but I rarely felt relaxed or at ease in the company of others.

In junior high a group of the most popular girls called each other every night to hash over the school day and gossip. My best friend was in this group and while I was comfortable talking with her, I felt awkward talking on the phone with anyone else. For example, the first and only time I talked on the phone with "Judy," I knew I was expected to speak with her for one hour or more. I ran out of topics after 10 minutes but continued having an awkward and strained conversation for the remaining 50 minutes before hanging up, sadly concluding, "I'm different. I don't fit in."

In high school, I played on the girls' softball team. I remember standing on third base yawning and yawning, trying to stay awake. It seemed strange to me, as I was not tired. Who yawns while playing a sport? I do, I reasoned, because I am different. Now I know I yawned from boredom and struggled to stay awake.

Even as an adult my differences were observed and questioned. When my five-year-old son injured his finger and came to me for comfort, I responded by putting a bandage on his finger but offered no words of comfort. He asked, "Why are you different from other moms?" When I took ballroom dance lessons years later, the same son, then a teenager, asked, "Why can't you remember the dance steps?" A neighbor once told me, "You're different." When I worked at a retirement community, a resident said, "You're different." I was keeping count.

Was I sensitive to being told I was "different"? You bet I was!

After being told and believing for many years that I was different, I finally learned why from Dr. Smith: My ADHD makes me different. I was the first adult Dr. Smith treated for ADHD, and at the time I wrongly thought, "I'm the only adult with ADHD in the United States." Dr. Smith surprised me when he said, "I'm envious of you. You get to start a whole new life."

I didn't feel that way. I just discovered I had a disorder, and he was envious of me? Trying to cheer me up? Nice try! Can't you do better than that? All I wanted to do was leave his office as quickly as possible, to be away from the space where my self-image—and my life—were destroyed.

I doubted Steve would be supportive. I used to joke that as a surgeon, he was completely willing to cut something out to make a person well, but he was totally against taking medication. I learned over time, and not just with Steve, that when a family member exclaims, "You don't have ADHD," they are saying they don't believe this disorder exists, they don't want you to have this disorder or they are fearful they might have it as well.

I was fortunate that Dr. Smith diagnosed my ADHD. Most physicians in 1992 did not recognize it in adults. If they were familiar with ADHD in children, they believed children outgrew it when they became adults.

The fifth Diagnostic and Statistical Manual (DSM-V), the standard classification of mental disorders used by mental health professionals in the US, was published in 2013. It was the first time that it included modified criteria for Attention Deficit Disorder in adults. The DSM-V calls it Attention Deficit Hyperactivity Disorder (ADHD), but when Dr. Smith diagnosed me, it was called ADD (with or without hyperactivity). I had it without hyperactivity. I now say I have inattentive ADHD. My primary symptoms are inattention, distraction, impulsivity, disorganization, and forgetfulness.

After being diagnosed, medication improved my performance and relationships. The counseling I received and the reading I did taught me about inattentive ADHD behaviors. I began using techniques for managing or minimizing their disruptive influence. I was improving but my emotions were complicated.

It surprised me when, a year after my diagnosis, I blurted out, "I've been in a grieving process!" I had been unaware of grieving until the words came out of my mouth. I was grieving the loss of my self-image. I thought I was a unique individual who did a few things differently from others, but this was a source of pride. Now I learned that what made me unique was a disorder, an aberration. What I thought was "special" made my life more difficult and the lives of my family and friends more difficult when they interacted with me.

In short, I had a disability.

As I realized how others might view me, I was ashamed. I was not "special." Instead, there was something wrong with me and everyone knew it. That is why I received negative reactions over the years from family, friends and colleagues, even strangers. It all came flooding back—my inappropriate actions, the people I offended and the mistakes I made. I felt less than others and this made me awkward and self-conscious. Even though my interactions and relationships improved after medication, another part of me wanted to withdraw from socializing.

I grieved for the life I lost. My entire life was less than it could have been. If only someone had known of my ADHD earlier. If only someone had diagnosed and treated me as a child, so much of my life would have been easier. ADHD seemed responsible for every setback or disappointment in my life.

Many adults with ADHD are angry when they look back on their lives. They have unhappy memories of being demeaned, criticized, and made to feel inadequate. They wonder why they were not treated with kindness, patience, understanding, and love. They wonder why no one figured out that there was something wrong. It would have made such a difference!

I doubted the truthfulness of Dr. Smith's comment, but as time went on and my life improved, I remembered his hopeful words and they proved true.

It took me three years after learning about Bruce's inattentive ADHD to accept that I had the same disorder.

It took me a year in treatment to overcome my grief and recognize improvements in my life. It took four more years to conquer most of my inattentive ADHD challenges.

This timeframe might sound daunting, but it should not. If you are reluctant to start your journey, accepting and managing your ADHD will make you more satisfied than you might believe possible.

Myth: ADHD is not a real medical disorder.

Fact: The American Psychiatric Association recognizes ADHD as a medical disorder in its DSM (Diagnostic and Statistical Manual of Mental Disorders)—the official mental health guidebook used by psychologists and psychiatrists.

CHAPTER TEN

The Murky World of Diagnosis and Treatment

ALL MENTAL HEALTH CONDITIONS—BIPOLAR disorder, depression, anxiety or ADHD—have no defining test. No lab test, no x-ray, and no physical examination reveals the problem. As Dr. Smith did with me in 1992, healthcare providers evaluate those with ADHD based on symptoms. One psychiatrist jokingly told me he could diagnose the disorder as soon as someone walked into his office and commented on his medical degrees on the wall. It is rare that anyone notices them, but an adult with ADHD will. This psychiatrist confirms his private diagnosis by taking a history, completing a rating scale and obtaining information from relatives. Another physician told me that adults who believe they have ADHD usually do.

The maladaptive behaviors of someone with this disorder are behaviors everyone has. Everyone is distracted, forgetful or impulsive at one time or another. What distinguishes someone with ADHD is the frequency and severity of the behaviors. Dr. John Ratey believes even a mild form of a disorder benefits from treatment but some physicians and psychologists disagree. They require the patient to show significant ADHD behaviors before they diagnose and treat it. The treatments include medication, cognitive-behavioral therapy and sometimes coaching.

When someone breaks an arm, the doctor and the patient recognize what's wrong, how to fix it and what an ideal recovery will be—full use of the arm. With a near-sighted patient the eye doctor determines what's wrong, what to do to improve the patient's sight and what result he seeks—20/20 vision or as close as possible. With many medical conditions the physician employs various tests, examinations and lab work to determine what's wrong, what to do to get the patient well and what wellness will look like.

Unfortunately, ADHD is not at this point. Many psychiatrists and primary care practitioners are not adequately trained to identify ADHD in adults or to treat it. It continues to be a challenge to make the diagnosis, determine the best treatment, and assess a favorable outcome. There is not one treatment that works well for every patient, and there is no clear idea of how a "treated" person should feel and act. No test proves our ADHD is cured or completely controlled. We don't immediately know which and how much medication best corrects our faulty brains and enables us to improve the most. The answers are hard to come by.

However, we know that medication is the most effective treatment for ADHD, provided we work with a physician to find the right medication at the proper dose. Sometimes this can be a two or three-month process. Approximately 20 percent of people with ADHD never find a helpful medication they can tolerate due to the side effects.

The public media promote the belief that too many clinicians err on the side of over-diagnosing ADHD. However, researchers believe at least 4.4% of the population have ADHD and Russell Barkley, Ph.D., an ADHD researcher, says we treat less than 3% of the population. One concern with over-diagnosing any illness is that it distorts society's expectations of what is "normal" and "not normal" and what requires medical intervention and what does not. *Are too many children diagnosed with ADHD when they are normally active or normally distracted?*

The media and the lay public wrongly believe that children with no ADHD are routinely (and incorrectly) diagnosed with it. In contrast to these views, experienced ADHD diagnosticians suggest that many youths with ADHD are undiagnosed because their providers cannot document the number of symptoms required by the DSM-V. Twenty-five years ago Dr. John Ratey wrote *Shadow Syndromes* in which, based on his clinical experience, he said many patients who met less than the full criteria for a mental illness still benefitted from treatment. More recently, Stephen Faraone, Ph.D., an ADHD researcher, published research showing that patients with fewer than the required number of symptoms may benefit from treatment.

Twenty-five years ago Dr. John Ratey wrote *Shadow Syndromes* in which, based on his clinical experience, he said many patients who met less than the full criteria for a mental illness still benefitted from treatment.

Some believe children or adults want this diagnosis to get school or workplace accommodations. Others question if adults are diagnosed so that they have an excuse for why they have not done well in life. Few people object to the seriously impaired person diagnosed with this disorder but the issue remains murky for mild or moderate cases. Is it a disorder or is it a mild disability? At what point does it switch—from someone being a bit impulsive, a bit disorganized and a bit inattentive—to having a disorder? When is the condition severe enough to warrant taking medication, usually for a lifetime? Again, these questions don't have definitive answers.

I ssues around treatment can become more heated than issues around diagnosis. The most helpful medications are psychostimulants that are controlled substances. If the medications we took were not controlled substances there would be less bad press. In the past 25 years the diagnosis of depression in children increased almost as much as the diagnosis of ADHD in children but it rarely receives terrible press. The stigma of treatment would be eliminated if our medications were not stimulants.

A desirable solution is an over-the-counter product that treats ADHD. This would eliminate the resistance to treatment and there would be less stigma to a diagnosis. Alas, no effective over-the-counter treatment is available. We continue to hear, "I won't give stimulant medication to my child!" although stimulants are some of the safest medications when taken as prescribed. The clinician and patient need to evaluate if the improvement in the person's quality of life outweighs any unwarranted negative beliefs about stimulant medication.

Stimulant medications are fast acting. Within a few hours of taking a pill the patient or, more typically, a family member will know if the medication makes a positive difference. There are several minor side effects such as loss of appetite and insomnia but these dissipate over time or resolve by changing the dose or switching to another stimulant. Although popular culture sometimes claims that stimulants cause youth with ADHD to become drug abusers, that is not true. Treatment with stimulants protects patients with ADHD from future substance use disorders. Eighty percent of patients who take a stimulant for their ADHD find it helpful.

For me the choice was easy. I loved my stimulant medication! However, for others it might not be easy. For them I recommend education about ADHD from reliable sources—not the mass media, not "concerned" family members, not nosy neighbors and not the sales agents of "alternative products." ADHDevidence.org is a reliable source of information.

Getting medication for ADHD is like getting a prescription for eyeglasses. If the prescription is not spot on your vision will not improve as much as it could. The same applies to getting the proper medication at the correct dose for treating ADHD. I tried the various medications and Ritalin, 10 milligrams taken three times a day, helped me the most. Another medication reduced more of my symptoms but made it hard for me to fall asleep. I learned not to focus on getting a perfect brain. My brain fitness goal became the same as my physical fitness goal: to be fit enough to perform well. My brain fitness goal was to manage my ADHD symptoms well enough to be content with who I am.

One woman was diagnosed and "treated" for her ADHD for three years. She took Ritalin, but she continued to have car accidents and procrastinate. She saw a different clinician who believed Ritalin did not help her enough. He switched her to Dexedrine and she immediately realized what her life could be.

A patient may be treated for ADHD but without comparisons with other medications, he may not be taking the medication that helps the most. When I was diagnosed only three medications, all short-acting, were used in treating ADHD. Today there are at least 30 with different delivery systems and lengths of effectiveness. However, not all treating clinicians are familiar with or comfortable prescribing many of the newer medications.

It is essential to see a clinician knowledgeable about ADHD, a clinician who works with the patient instead of dictating to them. Find a clinician who knows what to expect when the patient takes medication and who knows the same medication at the same dose does not work for everyone. The patient needs to recognize changes in his behavior. Sometimes he needs another person to help with this, as people with ADHD are poor self-observers.

Dr. Edward Hallowell, a psychiatrist and an ADHD expert, tells of a spouse who, after taking medication for two weeks, returned to the doctor's office with his wife. The husband said, "The medication hasn't made a bit of difference." Meanwhile, the wife sat there with an astonished look on her face. She interrupted, declaring, "It has made an incredible difference! And, sweetheart, if you stop taking it, I'm divorcing you!"

Sometimes the improvement with medication is dramatic and the person functions very differently than before. Other times, the changes are subtle. What the person does differently does not surprise her. We act in a way that feels normal so we do not find it unusual. Often we can't put our finger on what improved; we only realize our lives have become easier. I don't know what changes happen in Bruce when he takes his medication but I don't get angry with him on those days. On the days I get angry I ask, "Did you take your medication today?" His answer is always, "No."

What changes should you watch for when taking medication? Dr. Ted Mandelkorn, a Seattle physician, now retired, who treated children with ADHD said, and "ADHDers on proper medication improve their attention span, concentration, memory, motor coordination, mood and on-task behavior. They decrease daydreaming, hyperactivity, anger, immature behavior, defiance and oppositional behavior. Medical treatment allows intellectual capabilities to function appropriately."

He adds, "It is important to remember what medication does. Using medication is like putting on glasses. Glasses do not make you behave, write a term paper or get up in the morning. They allow your eyes to function normally if you open them. You control whether you open your eyes and what you look at. Proper medication for ADHD allows our nervous system to send its chemical messages efficiently. This allows our skills and knowledge to function more normally. Medication does not provide skills or motivation to perform."

"ADDers often complain of forgotten appointments, incomplete work, mistakes in written work, frequent arguments with a family member or co-workers, excessive activity and impulsive behaviors. With medication many of these problem behaviors dramatically improve. Patients successfully treated with medication typically go to bed at night and find most of the day went the way they had planned. If the medication prescribed is not significantly helping with most of these concerns ask to change the dosage or change to another medication. Medication is not the proper one if it relieves only one dysfunction, such as trouble falling asleep, but not any others."

After my diagnosis I took Ritalin three times a day, preferably 30–45 minutes before a meal. You are familiar with my memory challenges. Can you imagine how often I forgot to take my medication? I learned to keep a few pills at work. I had a second chance if I forgot to take a pill at home. Taking Ritalin was not "Wow! What a difference!" but slowly I got several things in my life under control.

Before medication, "I'll take care of it later" meant I would never get back to it. After taking Ritalin I slowed down and told myself, "This is a problem. You spend time every day searching for your keys, purse and watch. What are you going to do about it?" It was irritating to force myself to practice the new behaviors. I imagined what I wanted—a life where I spent less time stressed out, annoyed and disorganized. I made progress and was on a path to a higher level of performance but hated relying on medication.

I read *The Unquiet Mind*, Kay Redfield Jamison's account of living with bipolar disorder. She stayed in therapy because her therapist reminded her to take her medication. My situation was not as drastic but I wished I did not have to take medication. Then I learned about a treatment for ADHD that did not involve medication.

A psychologist in Tacoma was taking part in a study of Low Energy Neurofeedback Systems (LENS), which claimed to reduce or eliminate the symptoms of several disorders, including ADHD. Eager to stop taking medication I signed up as a participant. Before starting the neurofeedback treatments the psychologist required me to complete a Test of Variable Attention (TOVA). The TOVA is not used to diagnose ADHD but measures a person's impulsive and inhibiting behaviors and can evaluate the response to medication. The TOVA would also measure my response to LENS.

The TOVA is a sophisticated computer program. For 20 minutes, at one-second intervals, a tiny black box appears on a computer screen. The research assistant instructed me to push a button as soon as the black box appeared in the top half of the screen. I was not to push the button when the black box appeared anywhere else on the screen. The program recorded the speed and accuracy of my responses, whether my response times increased over time and if my errors likewise increased. It recorded if I made errors of omission (not pushing the button when I should have) or commission (pushing the button when I should not have). Then it scored my results.

The first time I took the TOVA, I was not on medication. I sat in a small, darkened room, staring at the computer screen. This was a test and

I wanted to do well. I sat up straight, ready to hit the button and stared at the screen, trying not to blink. For the next 20 minutes it was torture to stare at the screen. I wanted to look away, to gaze at something else, to do anything to break the monotony. The black boxes appeared so fast that, as much as I wanted to, I could not look away.

After five minutes of intense watching, I was deathly tired and wanted to close my eyes. I fought to stay awake by rocking back and forth, jiggling my legs, stamping my feet and talking aloud. The research assistant behind me noticed my bizarre mannerisms and wrote them down. But what could I do? I needed to stay alert. At the end of the 20 minutes I was physically and mentally exhausted but was satisfied that I did well. It was a tremendous effort but I thought I earned a perfect score!

The following week I retook the test, this time after taking my medication. I would be a smarter test taker. Instead of sitting hunched toward the screen and tightly clutching the button, I sat back in the chair and relaxed. I held the button in my left hand, rested my right hand on my lap and cleared away the pencils, paper and other items around the computer screen so there was nothing to distract me.

The TOVA started. The boxes appeared so slowly! Did they change the test since the last time? But they would not do that—this was a research project. Between each box's appearance my mind wandered yet I easily responded whenever they appeared on the screen. The TOVA was fun and I was convinced I was doing well. I stayed relaxed for the whole 20 minutes with no desire to glance away, no mental exhaustion, and no need to move my body to stay alert and focused. Wow! Taking medication for my ADHD makes a difference!

Imagine my surprise and dismay when I learned my scores the following week. A score of minus 1.5 or lower indicates ADHD. On the first test, without medication, I scored minus 7.5. The second time, on medication, my score was minus 5.7. There was only a minor improvement in my score. The difference was in how I experienced the two tests.

What did my low TOVA scores mean? Was I still significantly ADHD, even on medication? Was a minor improvement in my scores all that medication achieved for me?

Before the TOVA tests I was content with how I managed. Now I had questions: "Could I function better if I had a brain that worked better?" Steve told me to ignore the TOVA scores, and to focus on how I felt about myself, but I continued to wonder, "How much better can I be? What else can I try?"

Following my poor TOVA scores I increased my dose of Ritalin but quickly realized that raising my dose was not the answer. I functioned better during the day but woke at 3 am and could not fall back to sleep. I accepted that no medication would improve my TOVA scores. For this reason I became a willing participant in LENS and signed the paperwork that acknowledged the experimental nature of the treatment and the risks involved.

The psychologist's assistant ran the treatment sessions. He taped wires to various places on my head, changing locations with each session. I went twice a week for sessions and sat with my eyes closed while the assistant flashed a light at my eyes. I am still confused about the procedure but the goal was to increase my beta waves that make the brain wakeful and decrease my theta waves that make the brain less alert.

If I reported trouble sleeping after any session, the assistant made adjustments in the next session, which resolved my sleep problem. But after one session I was unable to sleep most of the night. When I went to my next session, the assistant left the practice and the psychologist ran the session; however, he was unfamiliar with the intricacies of the LENS protocols. He was unable to calm down my brain's wakeful state.

Eager for a treatment that got all of us off medications I had Bruce and Jackson try LENS. Today I am skeptical about the treatment. Even after 25 years, there is no research that neurofeedback helps and does no harm. Twenty-five years ago I was not wary. Eager to get off medication, I signed on the dotted line, no questions asked and signed for my sons as well.

While LENS did not "cure" my ADHD, there was enough recognizable improvement that I stopped taking medication. The downside was the disruption in my sleep. After spending sleepless night after sleepless night wandering the house at 1 am wide awake, I was utterly discouraged and regretted taking the treatment. Was a sleepless life now my fate? Going without sleep is hard on anyone, but even more so for someone with ADHD. Both Bruce and Jackson also have sleep problems to this day.

Because I stopped the neurofeedback, I never got the follow-up TOVA test to see if my scores improved. What else could I try? What else might help? I wished for a test that could show the presence or absence of ADHD in my brain. However, as my sleepless nights continued, I became fearful of trying any other treatment and became content in accepting that my ADHD was not wholly eradicated or cured. Consistent with my experience, neurofeedback is not an effective treatment for ADHD.

I saw a sleep specialist who recommended Remeron, a prescription medication. I took one pill and slept all night. I slept most of the following morning as well, and when I attended Toastmasters at noon, I slept through the meeting. The next night I took part of a pill but no matter what I tried, I could not find the right amount to take. Besides, Remeron made me ravenously hungry and stopped working after taking it for five days. The sleep specialist had me try a few other medications, but none helped.

We finally settled on Zolpidem, Ambien's generic form. It was over a year since my last neurofeedback session and my brain had calmed down somewhat. I fell asleep on 2.5 mg of Zolpidem, took another 2.5 mg when I woke up during the night and another 2.5 mg if I woke up a second time. This has been my routine for over 20 years. Ironically I traded taking Ritalin three times a day for taking Zolpidem three times a night. Ambien/Zolpidem has not become habit-forming for me although physicians warn about that.

Although progress has been made in the diagnosis of ADHD and today there are many effective medications for its treatment, we still have no way to determine which will work best for any given patient. Prescribers must use trial and error to find the best medication. We still do not know when people with ADHD have been helped enough to be all they can be. That knowledge awaits us someday in the future.

Myth: ADHD is an excuse for not trying hard enough.
Fact: People with ADHD try very hard to be successful, but their ADHD brain interferes with their ability to focus and work on tasks that are mundane, repetitive, boring, or require mental effort. People with ADHD struggle to accomplish the routine chores of life. It takes a massive mental effort for them to focus even on crucial tasks that are not novel, exciting, and interesting.

CHAPTER ELEVEN

Distraction and Inattention

S OMEONE WITH ADHD IS distractible, and often distraction combines with inattention. Sometimes I don't know which to blame, but it helps to understand the difference between these two behaviors and how they affect someone with ADHD.

For me *distraction* occurs when I should pay attention to one thing but get attracted to something else in my physical environment that is more engaging. For example, I attend a board meeting on Zoom but find that one board member talks at length about an unrelated topic. I get distracted and read the email on my iPhone.

Inattention is an internal event. I am still present at the board meeting but my mind goes elsewhere, often unaware that my mind is wandering. I think about what I will make for supper or what tasks I have to do after I leave the meeting.

For someone observing me distraction and inattention might seem the same. In both situations I am not present for the discussion. When I struggle with distraction the shinier, more attractive object pulls my attention away. With inattention my mind wanders away to a thought, image or memory. Something is said that creates an idea in my head. Someone mentions Hawaii and an image appears in my head about vacationing in a sunny place, and soon my mind wanders off in a million different directions although I have never left my seat.

Distraction has more to do with my physical environment and can vary with the situation. Imagine you are talking to me about the latest book you read, and I notice a ketchup stain on your sweater. I find it hard to focus on what you are saying because I wonder whether I should tell you. Once I notice my distraction I might say, "Could you please repeat what you just said? I missed part of it." Depending on how well I know you I might add, "Because I was distracted by the stain on your sweater."

Before I knew about my ADHD, I knew I could not talk to someone with the TV on at a normal volume in the background. The volume did not affect the other person's ability to be in conversation with me but significantly affected my ability to stay focused. Terry Matlen, an ADHD coach, once described ADHD distractibility as trying to watch a TV show in a house with all the windows open and swarms of mosquitos outside. You may be looking at the TV but the mosquitoes distract your mind. Or, as often happens with someone with ADHD, I notice something in my environment that reminds me of something I meant to do earlier but forgot to do.

I recently read a post on Pinterest that truly describes what a day was like for me before my diagnosis and I worked to improve my behavior:
   I decide to water my flower boxes.
   As I turn on the hose, I peer over at my car and decide to wash it.

I get the car keys from the house and notice unopened mail on the table.

I decide to read the mail before washing the car.

I put the car keys on the table, put the junk mail in the recycling bin under the sink and noticed that it was full.

I decide to empty the trash but think, "Why not pay the bills that came in the mail and put them in the mailbox when I take out the rubbish?"

I get my checkbook but it's out of checks. I go upstairs to get extra checks and see dirty dishes on my desk. I bring them downstairs and put them in the dishwasher.

On the counter above the dishwasher, I see the reading glasses I searched for yesterday.

I decide to put my glasses near the computer so I will know where they are when I need them.

Back at my desk, I notice the extra checks which remind me to pay the bills. I bring the extra checks downstairs and see the TV remote peeking out from the newspapers on the kitchen table. I know I will want it later when watching TV so I carry the remote into the family room.

And on and on. My day goes quickly.

At the end of the day:

The flower boxes aren't watered.

The car isn't washed.

The bills aren't paid.

I can't find my glasses when I want to read the newspaper.

I don't remember where I put the remote.

And I don't recall what I did with the car keys.

I am genuinely baffled when I try to figure out why nothing was done today. I was busy all day and I'm exhausted.

Here's a perfect example that I am still not free of ADHD distractibility. As I typed this Steve came to my office to ask why he has been waiting the last 20 minutes for me in the basement. He has finished fixing the exercise bicycle so that I can work out. Meanwhile I came to the computer for information on the broken bicycle part and instead became preoccupied with the Pinterest article I just quoted! I laughed as I handed Steve the article saying, "What this article describes is exactly what I've been doing! I started out searching for a bicycle part and now I am working on my memoir. I forgot about riding the exercise bike!"

In what circumstances would I be inattentive? Here is an example: You are talking to me about the latest book you read, going on and on, and I am not interested. Without being aware of it, I stop listening to you and instead wonder about what I have to do later in the day. Your uninteresting blather pushed my mind away to think about other things.

Does my mind wander to a magical place when I am inattentive? Do I have great thoughts? Not always but sometimes my best ideas just pop into my head. I astonished a friend when I told her about a solution to a problem we had discussed that came to me while I was making supper. Usually I don't think about something special when inattentive. I might remind myself of things I need to do and work out the order to do them or I might think about the weather.

Inattention is like internet surfing, starting at one website and then, 45 minutes later, having followed link after link, you are on a website on a different topic. Often, I wonder how I think about deer in our yard when I started out thinking about my friend in Australia. An image that might help you understand ADHD inattention is this: You are hiking on a hilly, rocky trail. Although signs along the way say, "It's important to stay on the trail!" you meander among the grassy fields that border the trail, lost in your thoughts.

Many people with ADHD need to keep their minds occupied. If they have nothing particular to think about, their fallback position is to worry. Worrying keeps our minds engaged and that makes us feel alive. I eliminated worry years ago.

Steve and I were leaving Allison for a few days to hike in the mountains of Malawi and I stayed awake most of the night before we left, worrying about things to tell the babysitter. For the night's worry and loss of sleep, I thought of only one more thing to say to her. That cured me of worrying.

If I fall into the trap and start churning the same thoughts repeatedly, I tell myself, "Stop. You've already thought about this and there isn't anything new to think about it. It's a waste of time. Repeating the same thoughts makes you feel bad and doesn't solve anything." Another effective way to stop churning thoughts is to take five slow, deep breaths. While taking those breaths, slowly look at your surroundings. If, after doing this, you continue to churn distressing thoughts, keep repeating the five breaths routine until your mind has shaken free.

When Steve has a faraway look in his eyes and I ask him what he is thinking, it amazes me that he says, "Nothing." I say to myself, "That can't be true. How can you not be thinking of something? You just don't want to share your thoughts with me." Then I realize that even though it is difficult for me to believe, he is genuinely not thinking of anything, and that is what most people do when they sit around with contented looks on their faces.

However, for me, it feels like I am always thinking.

Too much thinking. That is why some people with ADHD have trouble falling asleep. They lie in bed, tired and ready to doze off but cannot turn off their thoughts. Their minds are too full of thoughts. Usually I am tired by 11 pm but then ideas stimulate my mind and I am wide-awake.

The drawback of being confined by COVID, retired and no longer having a family to raise is that I have few things to think about. It was not my choice but my life became smaller. I ponder other people's thoughts through reading, viewing webinars and watching movies, but it's a poor substitute for the joy of juggling many ideas of my creation all day long.

Yet the COVID confinement got me to write this book which was a new and exciting challenge.

I reengaged with the ADHD community and updated my knowledge. I learned that children with inattentive ADHD were still under-diagnosed and adults with inattentive ADHD were often incorrectly diagnosed. I decided to start a non-profit organization with a mission to change that. The only way I persuaded myself (at 77 years old) to start the Inattentive ADHD Coalition was to ask myself, "If not you, who?" That convinced me to try.

After 10 years of complete retirement I now work about 30 hours a week (but who is counting?) for the Coalition. My mind is active. I have many ideas and am always thinking, which feels great.

Another aspect of my ADHD is that I could not have two thoughts simultaneously. If I thought about one thing and then thought about something else, I focused on the second thing and forgot the first. John Ratey, MD, an associate clinical professor of psychiatry at Harvard Medical School and an internationally recognized expert in neuropsychiatry, says that the inability of adults with this disorder to maintain focus is a key factor in their not improving, even after getting medication. This is why ADHD coaching has become a recommended part of treatment.

The coach keeps the client with ADHD focused on his goals (which is somewhat surprising when many ADHD coaches have ADHD themselves.)

Not sticking with something long enough to make a change rings true for me. Sometimes we shift focus to something more appealing because we lose interest in what we are doing. Other times we are interested and committed to our task, but we are called away to something else and forget to return to what we were committed to.

The first time I had two thoughts at the same time the novelty of it surprised me. After I started Ritalin, I was at work when visitors arrived for a facility tour. I told them I had to leave in thirty minutes to pick up my son at 3 pm. In the past I became engaged in giving the tour and, unnoticed, the minutes slipped by. But this day, after thirty minutes, I looked at my watch and told the visitors it was time for me to leave. I was pleasantly surprised and proud that I remembered my commitment.

Interruptions make me lose my focus. When I cook I need to be alone, with no conversation. Even when Steve asks how he can help, I get irritated instead of pleased. I can't drive and talk at the same time. If I drive and engage in conversation, do not hold me responsible for where we end up!

When I founded the non-profit organization ADD Resources, we invited national authorities to give presentations. For one conference I drove Dr. Daniel Amen, a psychiatrist, to the auditorium. I got engrossed in telling him about the challenges I had with Jackson. Dr. Amen startled me when he interrupted to ask, "Do you know where we are?" I looked around and sheepishly said, "No, I don't." (This was before cell phones and Google maps.) Luckily, a colleague was waiting for us on an off-ramp. When I noticed his car I breathed a sigh of relief and followed him to the auditorium. After that whenever Dr. Amen mentioned in his presentations that he was reluctant to get into a car driven by someone with ADHD, I knew he had me in mind.

Shortly after I married Steve we moved from Boston to Seattle. During my first year there I received four traffic tickets for moving violations, paid the fines, and the judge ordered me to attend driver education training. I joked, "It's true. Massachusetts has terrible drivers," but the actual truth was I drove without paying attention. The tickets and fines created anxiety in me when I drove which helped me to pay attention, but it was not a good solution. Since my first year in Seattle I have backed into cars in parking lots numerous times! My inattention caused these accidents.

Following one of my frequent car accidents, I called our insurance company to file a report. The agent turned on a recorder and asked a series of questions.

What was the make of the other car?

"I don't know."

Which car got to the intersection first?

"I did."

How many people were in the other car?

"I'm not sure."

Was there any damage?

"A bit of damage to her car. Not much."

Was anyone hurt?

"I don't think so."

How fast were you driving?

"Not fast."

I answered the questions poorly because I had not noticed what he asked about. My mind was probably on the song playing on the radio when the accident happened.

When I was an ADHD coach one client drove to see me from a town thirteen miles away. She told me she could not remember anything about her drive-in. Inattentive! I refrained from asking her if she was engrossed in a song playing on the radio. Adults with ADHD often drive fast; they find this is the only way they can attend to their driving.

New research about inattentive ADHD suggests that a slow processing speed often exists with this presentation, making me view a few of my challenges differently. It helped me understand why others laugh at a joke while I say, "I don't get it."

Years ago I learned that there's a difference between hearing and listening. When you are hearing your brain registers sound while with listening your brain comprehends what was said. Similarly, there's a difference between seeing and perceiving. With seeing, the brain notices something; with perceiving the brain gives meaning to what is observed. With a slow processing speed my brain does not perceive things quickly and, I believe it explains some of my crazy accidents.

In 2006, I backed our recently purchased van into a truck parked in front of our house. Yes, I saw the truck when I got into the van but my brain did not register its presence. What I told Steve in explaining the accident was, "That truck isn't usually there." Our van with less than 4,000 miles on it required $4,500 of repairs and needed to be in the shop for two weeks. Steve suggested I increase my medication.

Another time I needed to get to the ski bus by 7 am but was late. I saw the closed garage door, yet my brain did not register it. I got in the car, started it and backed into the garage door. I could not open it as it was dented. I home from skiing and we purchased a new garage door.

Another day when late for work I rushed out the front door and noticed that the boat trailer was attached to the van. I could not drive the van with the attached trailer but since it took Steve, Charles and Bruce to lift it off the hitch, I knew I needed help. I hurried next door, woke the neighbor boy, and asked him to help.

I said, "Peter, this will be difficult. It takes Dr. Hammer, Charles and Bruce to get the trailer off the hitch."

We crouched down and gave it everything we had. The trailer flew up in the air, light as a feather. Only then did my brain register that the boat was not on the trailer. Embarrassed, I said to Peter, "The trailer is difficult to lift only when the boat is on it."

Distraction and inattention are expensive problems. Besides damaging items I have lost possessions because I didn't pay attention when I put them down. If I have something on my mind I don't notice where I put things. My mind was occupied whenever we hosted conferences. I learned to wear a fanny pack to hold my camera, car keys and conference receipts so I would not put them down and lose them.

When I discover money in a coat pocket I consider it a lucky day. My discovery makes up for my annoyance when I could not find the money weeks or months earlier. I recently wore a coat I had not worn in several months and in a pocket I found a key I had given up for lost. The joy of discovery! Maybe I have too many coats! I do best with one purse so perhaps I should have one coat.

Bruce had an infection from an unknown source that traveled to his heart and damaged a valve. He had two open-heart surgeries, one in Tacoma and another a year later in Seattle but he continued to have a hole in his heart. Our last resource was the Cleveland Clinic, a mecca for open-heart operations.

I have hearing aids I rarely wear but I wore them to Cleveland. I wanted to hear everything the physician said after Bruce's surgery. The Cleveland Clinic supports family members in various ways—afternoon concerts in the lobby, incredible artwork throughout the hospital and free massages. They sponsor a shuttle to the Cleveland Art Museum, well known for its fabulous collection. One afternoon Steve and I toured the museum. I removed my hearing aids to wear their headset with the audio program. After leaving the museum I realized I did not have my hearing aids. They were somewhere in the art museum but I never found them.

On a hike through the Cotswold in England I put my credit card and driver's license in my jeans' pocket. During the hike I pulled them out unawares and dropped them. They were not there when we finished the hike and I did not know where they were. Why hadn't I taken care of my license and credit card? We planned to do the hike again the next day to search for them.

That night I called my son Charles in California and told him what had happened. He said a man from England posted to his wife's Facebook page that he found a credit card and license with the name Hammer and wondered if she knew the owner. Charles gave me the man's name and phone number and I called him. He lived an hour away from where we stayed. In the morning we drove over and retrieved my possessions.

For another vacation Steve and I were eager to start a two-week bike trip through southwest Wisconsin. We arrived at the Minneapolis-St. Paul airport with our tandem bike and two panniers. Before leaving the airport I hit the restroom. It was not until I was outside the airport that I wondered where I had left my fanny pack with blank checks, my driver's license, a credit card and my digital camera. It was back in the restroom with no possibility of retrieving it. Security allows no one through without identification and a boarding pass.

Steve had a credit card with him but it was the same as the one in my fanny pack. If I canceled the card or put a hold on it, he could not use it. He had an American Express card but we wondered if restaurants and hotels in Wisconsin accepted it. I thought my son at home could send me my passport so I would have an ID for the return flight. Then I worried, "What if my passport gets lost in the mail?"

Although I had little hope of recovering my fanny pack and possessions, I went to the airport's Lost and Found and made a report. It was Friday afternoon and Lost and Found was closed until Monday. I asked my credit card company to put a hold on the missing card.

I called Lost and Found on Monday and was told someone had turned in my fanny pack. Can you imagine my delight? We made plans to pick up the fanny pack in two weeks when we returned to the airport. Steve called the credit card company to take the hold off the card. The agent asked the fatal question, "Do you have the card in your possession?" Steve answered truthfully that we did not. The agent said, "We can't remove the hold if the card is not in your possession!" Yikes! We just made a colossal blunder.

Desperation made me bold. I called back to say my husband misspoke. I got the agent who talked with Steve and told her the card was in our possession. She said, "I don't believe you. We have a recording of your husband telling us it wasn't."

There was nothing we could do. We asked Lost and Found to send us the fanny pack overnight. I called the credit card company two days later to say the card was in my possession. A different agent, unaware of the recorded phone call, believed me.

Despite our inauspicious start it was a fantastic bicycle trip!

Isn't there a saying about God and fools? The first known use of this expression was in Harper's Magazine in 1856 where an article stated,

"A special Providence watches over children, drunkards and the United States. They make so many blunders and yet live through them; it must be they are cared for, for they take little care of themselves." It sounds like it was written with me in mind.

How did I react to each loss?

Disappointed.

Discouraged.

Diminished.

I have learned that with treatment disappointment and discouragement subside. It took longer to overcome my feelings of diminishment and shame but one of Eleanor Roosevelt's famous quotes bolstered me, "No one can make you feel inferior without your consent." I focused on not putting myself down when I did not live up to my expectations or what I thought were the expectations of others. I learned to accept myself, warts and all, which was easier once I had fewer warts to contend with.

Now I have better control over my troublesome behaviors. I know how I come across to others and adjust my behavior accordingly. I know I am forgetful and prone to distraction and I forgive myself. My disorder does not make me a lesser person. By learning about ADHD and being treated for it, I am all I was and have the potential to be even more. I am not a new model but an improved one with increased self-confidence and self-esteem. I am improved even though not ADHD-free.

Life is a continuing adventure that I face with confidence and optimism.

ADHD impairs people across the full range of intelligence, so yes, highly intelligent people can and do have ADHD.

CHAPTER TWELVE

ADHD and Social Niceties

THE REASON SELF-IDENTIFICATION OR self-diagnosis can be difficult for people with ADHD is that we typically lack self-awareness. I knew when I offended co-workers but did not always understand how or why. I was afraid to ask, worrying it would make them even more annoyed if they believed that the reason for their annoyance was evident.

For example, the secretary where I worked had an attitude whenever I asked her for something. I don't believe she acted huffy and put-upon with other employees. She did not sigh, grimace and shake her head with them as she did with me. She did not get up slowly to fulfill their requests, only with my requests. I wondered, "Is it this request? Or was it something I said or did much earlier that offended her and I have been in her bad graces ever since?"

I became reluctant to ask her for anything, even when she was the only one who knew where the copier paper was. If I had to guess why I annoyed her, it would be my forgetfulness of the simplest tasks. If

I didn't perform a task often, no matter how simple, I forgot how to do it. More than once I needed her to show me how to use the copier. More than once I asked her if she had a pen I could borrow because I had left mine in my office upstairs.

Medication can make us more aware of how others perceive us but it rarely eliminates the problem. I thought I had reasonably good relations with the admissions director when I worked at the retirement home. It was a shock to me when she wrote me a note at the urging of her therapist a few years after she retired.

"You often made me feel uncomfortable and inadequate. I'm relieved that I can finally write this note and tell you. I'm glad I no longer work with you."

What she wrote hurt me, but I put it out of my mind by telling myself, "She was too sensitive. She took anything I said too much to heart. I don't like everyone and everyone doesn't like me."

However, people with ADHD delude themselves when they believe, "I'm fine. It's my friends or work associates who have problems." When I got a less than stellar review from the manager of my multi-disciplinary team, I found it easy to dismiss what she said about my work because I did not respect her.

We justify why we did something a certain way and do not understand why others have a problem with what we did. For example, if I join a group collating the pages for a booklet and notice that they are doing it inefficiently, I might say, "This would be much faster if we laid the pages out this way." Then I take over, presuming that everyone wants to do the job more efficiently.

However, usually I am wrong and I impose my values on them. They had not asked me to make collating more efficient. They enjoyed the slow work pace that allowed them to chat with one another so they were resentful when I imposed a new system on them.

I recently volunteered to help at an organization and noticed that the staff person did not have a list of what she needed to review with new volunteers. Several items, like where to park the car and how to record my hours, were not explained to me. When I asked about these items days later she realized she had forgotten to tell me. That is when I suggested she make a list for new volunteers. She was irritated by my suggestion. Perhaps my tone of voice, a combination of impatience and irritation, led to a poor reception for what I thought was a helpful suggestion. Steve has often said to me in an irritated voice, "It's not what you say but how you say it." (Although I have not heard that remark from him for years. Progress! Yeah!)

The language of social niceties does not come naturally to me. Once I was at the bank with Jackson when he was about 12 and afterward he asked me why I was so mean to the teller. I didn't know what to say. I interacted with her in my usual way, not unpleasantly, just efficiently. The daily pleasantries of smiling and asking, "How is your day going?" take a conscious effort on my part. Often I find social niceties, such as "Have a wonderful day" or "Let's get together soon" to be stupid and meaningless. Why bother saying them?

I find it difficult to say things I don't truly feel or believe. Other times I am not immediately in touch with my feelings or thoughts so I don't express myself well in the moment. That might be why I prefer to communicate my thoughts in writing. Verbal communication requires a faster processing speed than writing.

Sometimes I feel like I never got the Owner's Manual. I miss essential information on how to operate in life. Often girls and women with undiagnosed ADHD learn to expertly cover up or hide their natural personalities to conform and fit in. It is believed that masking delays or prevents an ADHD diagnosis and erodes a person's self-esteem because, with masking, they lose a sense of self.

I had not heard of masking until this year, and because I lacked social awareness about what to do to fit in, I doubt I ever masked.

T his is a strange example that occurred years after I was diagnosed with inattentive ADHD. Still, it is when I was truly struck with the belief, "I lack basic information that other women, my comparison group, are born with. They instinctively know how to be socially correct and acceptable and what's more, they seem to enjoy it!"

I was hiking with friends at Mt. Rainier National Park and went to use the restroom. I noticed a woman's feet in the stall next to mine. Her feet were turned, not towards the door, but the back wall. I wondered, "What is she doing?" Then I saw only one foot on the floor and heard the toilet flush. "Oh! She pushed the toilet's handle with her other foot! How did she know to do that?" When I asked my friends about it, they were astonished. My hiking friends assumed everyone knew what I wondered about, everyone, that is, but me.

Here is another example. (Although I will sound dull-witted, I am committed to full disclosure.) One time a friend stopped by my house and we stood in the doorway chatting, then she left. Afterward I wondered, "Why didn't Mary come in to visit for a while?" Then, duh, I thought, "Because you didn't invite her in. That is what women do as well as suggest a cup of coffee or a glass of wine."

Another relationship problem that people with ADHD face is that we long for the intimacy that comes with deeper friendships but we do not understand or employ the expected steps to create those friendships. Caroline McGuire, M.Ed., says that adults with ADHD try to rush their relationships. We ignore the stages necessary for establishing an intimate relationship and overshare more than is appropriate. We frighten off those we want to befriend. Social niceties have their place in fostering lasting friendships and we ignore them at our peril. People with ADHD find engaging in the expected social chit-chat, the first stage in developing a friendship, boring.

Here are comments from adults with ADHD posted at reddit. com/ADD:

- Small talk can be profoundly dull. My brain wanders off.

- Yesterday I talked with a friend with ADHD about how typical conversations go. One person says his whole monologue and then the other person says her entire monologue. The monologue-ing gets so boring it's hard for us to stay engaged.

- We prefer conversations where people interrupt with interesting tidbits, making the conversation more engaging and exciting. Our preferred way of communicating is perfectly acceptable although there are settings where we need to reel in our enthusiasm and engage in more socially acceptable ways.

One winter's day I went cross-country with two new female friends. I was tired so I rested on the backseat of the car on the drive home while the other two women sat in the front seat and happily chatted the whole drive home. I listened, off and on, to their 90-minute conversation and realized, "I could never talk about those topics for that length of time and with so much interest." My following thought was, " . . . and I wouldn't want to."

I recalled a few luncheons where I needed to hold up my end of the conversation and realized I was exhausted after these luncheons without understanding why. Now I knew. Just like my experience taking the

TOVA when I was not medicated for my ADHD, maintaining a conversation that was not interesting was stressful and wore me out.

I don't have judgment about people enjoying light social conversation, but I don't have a judgment that it's not for me, either.

To give you a flavor of the kind of conversations people with ADHD find engaging, here is an example from a post on Reddit. Because the responses to the post are written, no one could interrupt, but in person, it is another matter. Interruptions are expected when we talk with each other as they add to the conversation's excitement, intensity, creativity and flavor.

Here is the post: "My boss who knows about my ADHD shows me the abandoned cellar at work and says, 'Explore this for me.'" Three photos of the cellar accompanied the post and the post received 630 comments. Here are a few of the comments that stayed on the topic:

- No fair! My ADHD only got me on Adderall! You get an abandoned cellar?

- Dang! My bosses have never found me a cool abandoned cellar to explore!

- Your boss knows how to harness an ADHD brain!

- Look! A box full of unlabeled booze and tangled Christmas lights!

- My fear of wound infections is battling my ADHD's desire to explore things.

- We have tetanus vaccines. Get yourself some unnecessary injuries!

- Oh God! Things to label AND things to untangle?? Sign me up!

And there were numerous unrelated comments inserted along the way about Edgar Allen Poe, the House of Usher, Armadillo sherry and its tastiness, spelunking, Ape caves in Washington state, asbestos, mold, dogs and wearing masks.

After over 400 posts, someone wrote, "Omg WAT!? I love this and I didn't know I needed it!"

Then the initial poster commented, "Well, that was a fun read through the comments! :) I wasn't expecting so much enthusiasm."

B eing socially appropriate is not easy for me. When I become engrossed in what I am saying, I don't perceive the other person's lack of interest. I recall a dinner Steve and I had with another couple at a restaurant in Seattle. It was our first time together and I openly talked about personal issues, such as family problems. I overshared. When I finished speaking, I expected the other couple to return with something equally revealing and personal. Instead they sat there with their eyes glazed and their mouths shut. The quiet at the table became awkward for all of us. It was not an evening to remember.

My lack of self-awareness made me unable to examine my actions and say, "This is ADHD behavior." However, when I looked at Bruce's behaviors, I realized I did many of the same things. The things he did that annoyed me were things I also did! When I analyzed my son's annoying behaviors, I understood how I annoyed others.

For example, he became argumentative when he wanted something I didn't want him to have, just as I "reasoned" with Steve why we should do something a certain way, i.e., the way I thought we should do it. When Bruce forgot a commitment he made or decided the commitment was no longer important to keep, he might or might not call to explain.

He believed it was no big deal that he let me down. Similarly, if I became overwhelmed with too much going on in my life (even though it was my fault I had too much going on), I expected those I let down to understand and forgive. I asked, "Why are you making it a big deal?"

These behaviors make us appear selfish to others, yet we never think of ourselves as selfish. Our priorities change and we do not understand why someone else has a problem with that. We believe, incorrectly, that it would not upset us if someone acted like that.

When I am with a group and have an idea about what the group should do, I have gotten feedback from Steve that I come across as forcing my will on the group. If they do not have any ideas about what to do, I will make suggestions. I don't feel like I am deciding for the group but Steve says it seems like I am.

When I observed the time-consuming ways that many decisions are made in groups, I realized I get impatient with obtaining input from everyone before proceeding. I believe this is why many people with ADHD prefer to work independently, make their own decisions or be in charge so they are expected to decide for others.

I have an impulsive tongue. I speak before I think.

Every Tuesday, unless it's raining, I bicycle with members of the Tacoma Wheelmen. We are a group of retired or semi-retired folks and our chief consideration each time is, "Where will we eat lunch?"

A few weeks back a younger person in excellent cycling shape joined us. When we commented on his fitness, he responded that he weighed 220 pounds two years ago and now he weighed 165. He became a vegetarian, he told us, because he had ulcerative colitis. At one point he mentioned his wife was Korean and that he ate kimchee, a spicy cabbage dish. That is when I blurted out, "That's what probably caused your colitis!"

I didn't realize this was an inappropriate thing to say. One club member immediately said, "Cynthia!" Another added, "I can't believe you said that." Not catching on, I defended myself: "No really, have you ever tried that stuff?"

Now, looking back, I ponder my faux pas. Why didn't I realize that this was the wrong thing to say? Why did I become defensive instead of immediately apologizing? The young guy never came back to ride with us. Were my comments the cause? What does everybody else know that I don't? And when will I learn?

Myth: ADHD results from bad parenting.
Fact: ADHD is rooted in brain chemistry, not discipline. How do critics explain that the same parents challenged to raise their child with ADHD are often model parents for their children without ADHD?

CHAPTER THIRTEEN

Step-by-Step Improvements

AFTER MY DIAGNOSIS AND taking medication, I implemented many coping strategies. Kate Kelly, co-author of *I'm Not Lazy, Stupid or Crazy*, calls the process "pulling oneself up by the boot-straps." It was difficult but I had to improve.

First, our house was chronically messy. How could my neighbors have so much time to visit each other and play with their children? In contrast, I spent all day indoors "working" and still had a messy house.

My solution for cleaning the house was to force myself not to leave a room until I had tidied everything in that room. I steeled my mind and did not permit myself to leave the bedroom until I made the bed and picked up the clothes. When washing dishes I compelled myself to stay at the sink. I longed to be elsewhere but fought these feelings. I had to have a clean kitchen before allowing myself to leave it. My *you-have-to-do-this-or-else-you-will-never-amount-to-anything* mentality worked.

Steve's insistence that we have a cleaning service once a week helped. For the longest time, I resisted. I was home all day, and I couldn't keep

the house clean? I thought hiring help was further proof of my inadequacy, but once free of the tedious, repetitive tasks of housecleaning,
I maintained enthusiasm for other, more interesting household chores.
Once we had the house cleaning service and my self-esteem did not rely
on how well I kept our home, I found delegation to be the ultimate
coping technique.

It was a lengthy process but I created "homes" for our possessions
and forced myself to return items to their "home." Between the cleaning
service and putting things promptly away where they belonged, our
house slowly became presentable and a calm retreat.

I read many books on organizing and slowly put the ideas in place.
I was tired of getting dressed to go somewhere only to discover my
outfit had a spot, had a button missing or needed hemming. I rushed to
put on something else, only to find out that it, too, had a problem that
made it unpresentable. I was already late, and not finding something
to wear made me even later. My anxiety soared, and my self-esteem
plummeted. I tried on one item of clothing after another, rushed to
the iron or sewing machine or gave up and wore the outfit as it was,
hoping no one noticed.

It amazes me how far I have come since then. I continue to maintain
the tidying-up habit. When I am ready to leave the house and see the
breakfast dishes on the counter, I put them in the dishwasher. Coming
home to a tidy kitchen cheers me. When the bed is made and the soiled
clothes are in the hamper, it gratifies me. When all the groceries are put
away, it pleases me and if I come home to a tidy house, it makes my day.

I have a board in my closet with cup hooks where my necklaces hang,
my scarves are neatly folded in a clear plastic box and unmatched socks

are discarded. Everything in my closet is ready to wear. The frantic and pathetic dash to get ready is gone and I don't miss it. Now the excitement and adrenaline rushes in my life come from fun, esteem-building activities.

When I started work as a discharge planner in the hospital, my primary concern was preparing dinner for my family. I mentioned my concern to my co-workers and it astonished them. Apparently, they did not have a problem with meal preparation but for me it was a significant obstacle. I thought about what to make for dinner when it was dinner-time and rushed to the grocery store. How could I prepare dinner for 6:30 pm if I didn't get through work until 5 pm?

Again, a change was in the works. It was like death to sit and plan the week's meals every Saturday morning, go to the grocery store and buy what was needed, but after I experienced the difference these changes made, it motivated me to make them part of my skills toolbox.

I developed the list-making habit many years ago but often lost the list and needed to make another one. Then I would forget items that were on my earlier list. I solved the problem by creating lists in a booklet in my purse.

I learned to plan my errands. Before leaving the house I made a list to make sure I had what I needed to make the errands successful—a sample screw when I needed to find four more, the light bulb to replace the one in the refrigerator, a swatch of fabric I wanted the paint to match. If I were buying window shades I would bring the window measurements to the store. My earlier self would have been buying shades, deep in discussion with the salesperson, without knowing what size was needed.

I used the phone before going in person. Did the store have what I needed? Was it in stock? Could they hold it for me at the checkout counter? Incorporating these changes made my life easier and made me feel competent.

Often people with ADHD do not put something away because we have not created a place for it. Sometimes we do not put things away because we are too busy to do it right then. We tell ourselves, "I'll do it later," but then the tasks pile up and overwhelm us. Our possessions are in disarray but we do not want to deal with them. As the days pass by we get used to our mess. Still we are ashamed to have someone visit our home or office and see our mess.

I watched a friend wipe up a spill on her kitchen floor. She got out the spray bottle and a cloth and wiped the spill away. Then she left the cloth and spray bottle where she used them and walked away to do something else. I said nothing but thought, "This is how it happens, one misplaced item and then another until the entire house is a mess."

There were many items I didn't put away: my coat on a chair, my purse on the kitchen counter, a book on the dining room table, the unopened mail on the kitchen table, and the newspaper scattered on the living room carpet. Without trying, someone with ADHD quickly creates chaos. Think of the mother who follows a toddler around, saying, "All I do all day is pick up after him." Unfortunately, people with ADHD do not have mothers who follow them around. We must learn to do this for ourselves if it is going to get done. A wife or a husband of a spouse with this disorder may assume the "mother" role, but this spells trouble for their marriage if they were not expecting an extra child in the family.

With a Germanic background, Steve is fond of saying, "A place for everything and everything in its place." Can you imagine how often he said that around our house? Fortunately, he is a tolerant person and I adopted his slogan (except for the pile that mysteriously grows on the kitchen counter, no matter how much I discourage its existence). If articles are left out during the day I cruise the house to tidy up before bed. How reassuring to wake up to a house where "alles ist in ordnung!"

My commitment to completing a task once started was especially helpful when cooking. When I made breakfast for my family I typically put the slices of French toast under the oven's broiler, walked away and forgot them. Another breakfast was ruined. Or I would start dinner, remember something to do in another part of the house, dash off and forget about dinner. Out of sight, out of mind—until the smoke alarm went off!

I forced myself to stay in the kitchen until the meal was ready. I found things to do while waiting—set the table, wash a few dishes, study recipes, and make a shopping list. Keeping the stove in sight reminded me, "You're cooking dinner!" I set the timer. If I became involved in reading the newspaper, the timer alerted me about the cake in the oven: another little but important improvement.

My mother-in-law was a clean-as-you-go cook—I could never tell a meal was even in preparation! When I finished preparing dinner dirty pots, pans and utensils covered every available space. Our kitchen never had enough counter space. I read about a homemaker who stuck her dirty dishes in the oven to get them out of the way and thought, "What a useful idea." I used to believe it was more efficient to clean the entire kitchen after the meal but I learned to be a clean-as-you-go cook, and it makes a world of difference. Breaking tasks into small, achievable parts helps people with ADHD not to get overwhelmed.

When preparing a meal I break cleaning the kitchen into separate tasks. I clean as much as I can while cooking and finish cleaning up after we have eaten. Before, when we had company for dinner, I saw the piles of dishes, pots and pans and headed to bed. I thought I would deal with the mess in the morning but I didn't want to deal with it then either. Now I run one load in the dishwasher and soak several items in the sink while we linger over dessert. I finish cleaning up after the company leaves.

Cleaning up became easier as there was less to do. It helps that my older friends leave by 9:30 pm.

Training myself consistently to put my credit card back in a specific place in my wallet was more challenging than training a seal to balance a ball on its nose. It took all my focused attention and commitment, which I did not have before medication to create this habit. I was motivated by remembering my confusion and shame when I got to the checkout and did not have my card, holding up a line of people as the cashier gave me a long, consoling look while I frantically searched my purse and wallet. Was it in my pocket? Was it loose in my purse? Had I left it in the car? Was it at the last place I shopped? Often I left the store without making a purchase.

The time spent hunting for my credit card added unproductive hours to my life. I was anxious and ashamed, not knowing where it was. I was not taking care of something essential. With effort I acquired the habit of putting my credit card back in its assigned place in my wallet. What a difference this minor change made for me. I have not personally tested this idea but someone told me it takes 30 repetitions to acquire a habit. He wanted to put his keys and wallet in the basket by the front door as soon as he entered the house so, I'm not joking, he went in and out of his house 30 times in a row, putting the keys and wallet in the basket on each trip.

Another strategy I developed was to have envelopes and deposit slips in my desk at work so I mailed my paycheck to the bank as soon as I received it. Before I developed this strategy I often misplaced my paycheck. A few times I had to ask my employer to reissue it.

Next I hyperfocused on putting my keys in their assigned place in my purse. I practiced until I always put them there when out and about but I often neglected to return my keys to my purse after entering the house. I might put them down anywhere. I practiced over and over—put the keys in my purse, put the keys in my purse, put the keys in my purse! I eventually learned. Not only do I have a special place for my keys in my purse but I have a special place in the front hall closet where I always— well, almost always—hang my purse when I arrive home. I no longer hunt for my keys or purse when I need to go somewhere.

Having my car keys readily available helped me achieve another of my goals, getting to places on time. The ADHD brain is activated when under stress. Adrenaline kicks in, which makes our brains work. When it's time to leave we think of things to do and we are motivated to get them done. We tidy the kitchen make the phone call we put off or feed the cat. Our last-minute activities make us late. With medication my brain was awake so I no longer needed the stimulus of running late.

I committed to getting to appointments and meetings on time. I wanted to be a prompt person as an on-time person is considerate and in control of her life. I developed a realistic sense of time. How long did it take to shower and get dressed? How long did it take to drive to certain parts of town?

Previously I miscalculated how long a trip would take. I knew the drive to the YMCA took five minutes but I did not include the time to get in the car, back out of the garage, park at the Y, rush inside and put on my gym clothes. Once I understood why I was late, I corrected my faulty thinking. Before medication I never took the time or had the interest to figure this out. Now I prefer to arrive early and wait rather than be late.

In the past when a project excited me I immediately started it. Soon my enthusiasm faded when I realized the project was a substantial undertaking, complicated and time-consuming. I had not thought it through. I had not thought at all!

I am still upset about the ski rack I tried to make for my sister's family. With much gusto, I started but I didn't finish it in time for Christmas. It was not turning out as I hoped so I lost interest. Her family did not get a present that year and the ski rack is now a tool rack in our garage. Like most adults with ADHD I have several "unfinished masterpieces."

A co-worker gave me this advice: Before starting on a project list everything that is required—the time, people, resources and materials. Think through the steps to completion. Often thinking about the project in this way dulled my enthusiasm. I was not excited about it once I realized all the work required. People with ADHD have countless ideas and remarkable enthusiasm and energy when starting a project, but sadly, our list of accomplishments is short. We are powerhouses at starting and terrible at finishing. Now I was on a new path, a warpath, to finish everything I started. No more impulsive decisions!

People with ADHD swing between being bored and being overwhelmed. It is hard for us to find the middle ground. Not putting off boring tasks is a particular challenge. Not being overwhelmed by all there is to do is an immense challenge as well. It's not until we become reflective (which I became after I took medication) that we realize putting off the tedious tasks is counter-productive. It causes too many tasks to pile up.

Procrastination is a common problem for people with ADHD. I lost the diamond out of my engagement ring because I never took it to a jeweler for regular inspections although I meant to. One day the prongs, which hold the diamond, scratched me. I looked down and the diamond was missing. Steve replaced the ring when a local jewelry store went out of business. I liked the Marquette diamond ring more but did not take better care of it. I never had it professionally evaluated and, you guessed correctly, one day the diamond from that ring went missing as well.

Recently I returned from visiting Charles and his family in Folsom, California. As I lay in bed I thought, "I must unpack my suitcase." Then I reflected on my return from past trips when I never had that thought. Unpacking was boring and a person with ADHD cannot tolerate boredom. I used to say, "I'll do it later" but now I knew that meant, "I don't want to do it!"

We are unconscious of this thought pattern. We wish the dreaded task magically disappeared because we do not want to deal with it. In the past when I did not unpack, weeks slipped by while I continued to rummage through my suitcase for the things I needed. Now I know that is not helpful. I don't unpack my suitcase with relish but unpacking it makes me feel better about myself. The bedroom looks better and the articles I need are in their usual place. I have to unpack sometime so why not now? It takes less than 10 minutes!

I used to put things off until later and when "later" came the task was still there waiting for me. "Doing it later," meant the chore became harder to do. A part got lost, the instructions were misplaced, the paintbrush dried out, or the wet laundry became mildewed. How often have we said those four brief words, "I'll do it later," only to rue the day? Why didn't we complete the task when we first needed to do it?

There are many mundane tasks a person with ADHD finds a challenge to complete—folding laundry, matching socks, opening the mail, paying bills, filing paperwork, hanging up clothes, and the list goes on and on. As much as I dislike it, I do these tasks now, not later, forcing myself to pursue a better course of action.

When I told a friend that life was mostly a question of luck, she said, "Luck and excellent choices!" I keep trying to make excellent choices.

To prevent getting overwhelmed, break tasks into manageable, bite-size pieces. Although it seems efficient to wait until the end of a project to clean it all up, we are too tired or overwhelmed by then. Like with cooking, clean up as you go along and put nothing off. Do what you can when you can.

A time management guru advises doing a task immediately if you can do it in less than three minutes. I have adapted his advice. If I can do a task in less than five minutes, I do it now. If not now I don't know when and I will forget it needs to be done. It takes effort to get started on a task I don't want to do. We must trick ourselves into starting. I may want to clean up my desk but the sight of it overwhelms me and I can't get started. However, if I break the chore into pieces, I fool myself into starting: "I will only clean this one drawer," but once started, I clean the whole desk.

When returning to a task it takes time for me to figure out where I left off because I rarely remember. Before I start on what's left to do I must review what I completed so I will not duplicate my work. Last year I paid quarterly taxes to the state twice because I forgot I had already paid them. To avoid mistakes like that, if I cannot complete a task in one session, I commit to finishing it soon. I write reminders about what I need to do so that I will remember. I break tasks into manageable parts and create commitments.

When we had company for dinner I was revved up as the clock approached 6 pm. Would my dinner guests arrive before I was ready? Will I be in the kitchen cooking when the doorbell rang, or will I be in the shower or getting dressed? It never was a question of if I was ready and waiting. I asked Steve to help me with the last-minute, hurried preparations but the frenzied activity which produced adrenaline in me produced anxiety in him. He said, "You can't have friends over again if it means a last-minute rush." Having deadlines gets people with ADHD into action but often at the last minute and in a slap-dash manner.

I changed. Instead of doing everything on the last day and in the final few hours I cleaned the house the weekend before, planned the meal and bought the groceries several days in advance, set the table and prepared much of the meal the day before and did the final preparations on the day of. I was ready and waiting when the guests arrived. No last-minute surprises, no hectic finish. I was organized but missed the excitement—the busyness, the commotion, my feeling of being "alive."

I did not like calm and flat. Dare I say it bored me without a last-minute juggling act? I missed my adrenaline rush and went through withdrawal. It took several dinners before I appreciated my new way of functioning. I learned to value being calm and in control and to enjoy being ready and rested when guests arrived. I still love adrenaline but seek it in other activities—such as riding my bike fast down hills, skiing on challenging terrain or learning new skills.

Does it sound like my life is perfect and ADHD is no problem? No way! It is an everyday struggle but recognizing and labeling my behaviors is an effective tool for managing my disorder. If something is a problem for me now I am confident I will solve it with ingenuity and determination. I give my problems the old one-two—ADHD creativity and ADHD perseverance—and continue on my journey by correcting my small but troublesome behaviors. I make progress despite the setbacks.

ADHD may co-exist in varying degrees with depression, general anxiety disorder, post-traumatic stress disorder, bipolar disorder, panic disorder and substance abuse.

PART FOUR

At Last, the Me I Was Meant to Be!

CHAPTER FOURTEEN

How Long Does It Take to Heal?

FOR THOSE RECENTLY DIAGNOSED what I have to say next might discourage you although I don't mean it to. Healing from ADHD is an exciting growth experience. We have the chance to become the best we can be. But no matter what, healing takes time.

Dr. Oren Mason says, "A lifelong transformation begins with diagnosis and proper medication." As mentioned before, medication never does the entire job of ADHD healing. Medication helps us improve our lives but it will never make us non-ADHD. It took me five years to heal emotionally. Still, as Dr. Mason explains, "There is no end to the learning potential that blossoms with treatment, both in executive functions and emotional self-management."

The first year after my diagnosis I was depressed; I spent the following years conquering my depression by improving my life. I believe I am now "healed" from my ADHD even though I still have it. We are healed when we are content with who we are, despite having ADHD.

Immediately after my diagnosis I withdrew from people around me. No one could understand how I felt, believing I was the only adult with ADHD in America. Then I found a book, *Attention Deficit Disorder in Adults* by Lynn Weiss, Ph.D. In the book's resource section, she listed Lisa Poast, a woman with ADHD in Bellingham, Washington. I called Lisa and we talked and talked. Lisa remembers how upset and shell-shocked I was to be diagnosed with inattentive ADHD. It was life-saving for me to connect with someone who shared my experiences. I could talk to Lisa about my triumphs and my setbacks. No matter how much progress we make there are always setbacks.

Last week my ADHD surfaced with a vengeance and many behaviors that I thought were under control returned! What was going on? Why was I back in a disorganized office? Why did I lose items that were in my hand only moments before? Where was the list I made? Why did I forget the items I wanted to purchase and spend an hour wandering around Home Depot, hoping to spy what I needed to buy? Why did I waste an hour browsing when I had many pressing chores? I was overwhelmed, attempting to do too much.

I still struggle to keep my focus only on the things I value. Too often people with ADHD are scattered. We find too many things appealing; too many ideas pull us in many directions. As a result we do not spend our time on what we truly care about. ADHD is like being in a television store with 50 TVs, each tuned to a different channel. You are expected to watch just one of those televisions but that is impossible. Medication reduces the number of TVs but learning to focus only on a few TVs is also essential.

Knowing my priorities and focusing on them is necessary to maintain balance. New, exciting ideas always occur to me but I evaluate them. Is this a priority? Does it contribute to my mission in life?

What enabled me to develop a focus for my life was writing my mission statement as recommended in *The Seven Habits of Highly Successful*

People by Steven Covey. What did I value? Who do I admire and for what reasons? What did I want to achieve? How did I want to achieve it? It took several months to ponder these questions. Learning my priorities was a lengthy process.

I kept putting off writing my mission statement. Finally, I wrote my mission statement when we flew to Boston. Sometimes we can only get ourselves to do something by ensuring there are no other alternatives. (As an aside, I recently heard about a person with ADHD who flew to Japan and back so that he could write the draft for his book. But the most creative idea I heard for staying in place until the job got done was a man who installed a seat belt on his office chair.) Once I started, my mission statement was easy to write. It surprised me how simple my mission was: to value my family, to focus on wanting close relations with my children when they became adults and to help adults with ADHD. Going through the thought process and writing the statement clarified what was meaningful to me and allowed me to say no to activities that were not part of my mission.

Besides "a place for everything and everything in its place," another slogan became my maxim: "You can do anything you want but not everything." Together these slogans keep me focused. I know my priorities; I know what is important to me. I accept that I don't have the time or energy for everything and have to pick where I put my effort if I want to be successful. My life is fulfilling when I accomplish things and when I complete what I start in a way that makes me proud.

This kind of focus earlier in my life would have helped me have fewer injuries as a child and as an adult. I never thought ADHD contributed to my injuries but research shows that adults with ADHD are accident-prone because of their inattention, hyperactivity or impulsivity.

I have injured almost every body part at least once. One early injury to my left knee eventually led to getting a total knee replacement when I was 50 years old.

During one of my college spring breaks my mother encouraged me to go skiing by myself and even loaned me her car. I went to Mount Snow in southern Vermont where I met two people to ski with, Jay and Bill. They were better skiers and I foolishly tried to keep up. When they skied over a jump I followed and fell when I landed. I injured my left knee and could not safely drive home. Bill drove me home in my car while Jay followed in his.

Dr. Wheeler, our family doctor, diagnosed a torn anterior cruciate and put a plaster cast on my leg. I returned to college with crutches and limited mobility, plodding up and down stairs to classrooms and back to the dorm. If I tried to go faster it only caused problems.

A student in my dorm wore steel braces on her legs. She used crutches and walked slowly wherever she went. When I observed her I thought, "How hard it must be to walk slowly all the time. How does she have the patience for it?" I did not have patience. I had my cast on for six weeks. With two weeks left I could tolerate it no longer. I stepped into the shower and turned on the hot water, hoping to dissolve the cast. I was unsuccessful. I could not get the cast off and it was not worth keeping on. I went home and Dr. Wheeler sawed it off. He had known me for years and did not express surprise at my impatience.

I overcame or minimized many of my troubling behaviors with coping or compensating techniques but other behaviors continue to trouble me no matter what I do or how hard I try. (Now my ADHD behaviors usually bring humor and laughter.) Sometimes I ask myself, "How could

I be so dumb when I'm not even blonde?" (Sorry, I could not resist.) I kept these dumb behaviors hidden for many years. Now I roll with the ADHD punches because I have enough areas where I function well.

If my ADHD rarely shows because I compensate well, why did it reappear with a vengeance last week? I was stressed. I had three significant deadlines and my brain could not handle them. Dr. Hallowell says, "About the worst thing someone says to an ADHD child or adult is, 'Try harder.'" Trying harder turns off our frontal lobes. I can practically feel my brain become scattered when I have too much to cope with. Perhaps we can manage only a certain number of balls in the air at one time. When our juggling becomes too complicated, the balls come crashing down.

This happened to me recently. After working for hours to perfect the materials for an innovative project—ADHD Skill-Building Tele courses—I screwed up the whole thing by sending emails to the wrong people with the incorrect dates and times. I wanted to shout in frustration and rage, "I hate having ADHD!" I am not a detail person. Why do I keep ignoring this knowledge and not carefully proofreading something before I send it? Why don't I ask someone to review my work instead of sending it without a final review?

Overcoming the impulsivity of ADHD has its challenges. Dr. Hallowell says that impulsivity can lead to creativity but impulsivity gone wrong? I don't want to think about it. Against my better judgment, here are some examples:

I used to wear contact lenses. Now I have permanent lenses after cataract surgery. But when I lived for three months in Wenatchee, Washington where almost every day is sunny but windy, I wore contacts. I rubbed my eye when playing tennis and my left contact lens fell on the court. I could not find it and immediately had the not-so-great idea: "I'll put my other contact lens on the ground. It will help me figure out what the missing lens looks like and I'll find it."

You guessed it. I lost both lenses.

We have a short hill, five feet in height and 100 feet long, that separates our yard from our neighbor's. Along this short hill is a rock garden. If I saw weeds to pull after I got home from work, I climbed into the rock garden in my best clothes, nylons, and high heels. I just could not stop myself from pulling those weeds.

Our house always has an area that needs touch-up painting but I never change into painting clothes. I always believe, "This time will be different. I will not get any paint on my clothes. It's such a little area to paint." A day or two later I notice paint spots on my best, but now ruined clothes. I don't take time to put down masking tape when I paint the molding that abuts the flooring.

You can guess the result.

My most expensive impulsive paint job was spilling a quart of paint on a loaned Oriental rug. We took the rug home to decide if we wanted to buy it. I tripped going up the stairs and the can of cream-colored paint flew out of my hands and landed upside down on the rug. No hiding that mistake. I have never been more embarrassed, especially when the storeowners came to inspect the damage. Thank goodness, our insurance paid for it. (Sometime after I was browsing through the insurance company's magazine and saw an article that gave an example of why people would want homeowner's insurance: spilling paint on an oriental rug.)

I have reduced my inattention, distractibility and impulsivity with the help of medication and learning from past mistakes but no treatment has improved my faulty memory. Forgetfulness is one aspect of my ADHD I have not overcome and it continues to create difficulties for me. I often had trouble finding my locker at the YMCA.

One day after swimming in the pool I went to my locker, opened it, and was shocked to find it empty. I immediately thought, "Someone stole my gym bag, clothes, towel and hairbrush! Who would want them? How am I going to get dry? How can I get dressed to go home?"

I searched the adjoining lockers but did not find my gear. However, one nearby locker had a lock on it. Recently I started using a lock but I didn't remember putting on a lock that day . . . and that lock did not look like mine . . . or did it? I tried the combination, which I was pleased to remember. The locker opened and there was my gear. Lucky day! Now I have learned to really, really, really notice my locker number.

Once, I made a blueberry pie for expected company. For the crust I combined flour and shortening in the bowl and then could not remember if I added salt. Three ingredients and I was in over my head! Did my body remember taking the salt from the shelf and pouring it into the measuring spoon? I could not remember. Impulsively I added a teaspoon of salt and then tasted the mixture. Was it too salty? You probably can guess the answer.

One of the depressing aspects of having a poor memory is not remembering people or events from my past. When I attended my 25th high school reunion and former classmates said hello, I had no memory of them or the events they discussed. Our high school class was fewer than 250 students and I spent many years with the same people. My sister speaks of things that happened when we were growing up and I ask in surprise, "Did that happen?" My treatment for ADHD did not improve my memory.

I developed the non-profit organization ADD Resources for adults with this disorder. Our office phone had two rings, one for the phone and another for the faxes. No matter how often I told myself not to answer the phone when it rang for a fax I picked it up. If the phone rang again a few minutes later for a fax, I picked it up again. Aargh!

I write the simplest things down because, as soon as I look away, I forget or I am not confident I remembered correctly. When I worked as a geriatric social worker at the retirement community, I joked that my brain was the three-ring notebook I carried. Without my notebook I was clueless. Now I use "Notes" on my iPhone for the same purpose.

After two years as the volunteer treasurer for a local non-profit where I made weekly bank deposits I memorized our twelve-digit bank account number after writing it down over 50 times. Progress! A friend who remembers a recipe after making it once amazes me. I made pancakes each week for my family and always looked up the recipe, unsure how much milk and flour it required.

Forgetfulness hits me in the face in the worst situations. Hiking in Europe I misplaced my passport. I was sure (as sure as I am of anything). I put it in my backpack but it was not there when I looked. We were on a ten-day hike around Mont Blanc. Worrying about where I left the passport made it difficult to enjoy the hike. Six days into our hike it appeared. It was wedged in the top of my backpack and hiking worked it loose.

At one conference, I experienced a major "ADHD moment." I was out to lunch when I was scheduled to present. Thankfully, the conference organizer found someone to present in my place and took my absence in stride for he, too, had ADHD. His motto, which I have used since, is, "If you're going to laugh about it later, you can laugh about it now." Having perspective can make some problems insignificant. If we imagine how a current crisis will appear in the future we deal with it better in the present.

Another of my memorable forgetful moments happened when we hosted Dr. Hallowell at our annual conference. For convenience the conference crew stayed in a Seattle hotel on Saturday night instead of returning to Tacoma. After the day's sessions we returned to the hotel to rest and relax before going to dinner. We agreed to meet in the lobby at 7 pm. After resting for a while, I went to shower and took out my contact lenses. I forgot their container at home but this was not a problem. I put both lenses in a glass of water. Since the lenses have the same prescription, it did not matter if they got switched. When I stepped out of the shower, I noticed an inviting glass of water on the sink and drank it.

Fortunately, I brought my eyeglasses. No one at dinner asked why I wore them.

Myth: ADHD affects only boys.
Fact: Children and adults can have ADHD regardless of gender, although boys are more likely to be diagnosed than girls. Girls typically have the inattentive type of ADHD, which is more challenging to recognize. Males and females with inattentive ADHD often are misdiagnosed with anxiety or depression.

CHAPTER FIFTEEN

The Power of Positive Self-Talk

D R. HALLOWELL SAYS PEOPLE with ADHD need to engage their minds to feel alive and that life is worth living. When our minds aren't engaged in an exciting or creative activity we launch into worry. I am not a worrier but when my mind is not engrossed in a stimulating activity, my life is flat. Many with ADHD are dysthymic—in a mild, chronic state of depression—without realizing the cause is their unengaged mind.

I feel overwhelmed and irritable with too many irons in the fire; with too few, life is dull. I cannot tolerate boredom! I get into action by doing something or too many things that interest me. I swing between being overwhelmed and underwhelmed, trying to find the right balance. Someday, perhaps, I will figure it out.

Inconsistent or variable performance is one reason people with ADHD have low self-esteem, despite doing extraordinary things. Because we perform inconsistently, we do not know what we can take credit for. Not understanding why we are successful sometimes and unsuccessful other times makes us lack the confidence to repeat our successes. When we do something well, we think, "It's a fluke." I overcame my feelings of inadequacy when I consistently performed well in a variety of situations. I counted on myself and people relied on me but this change took several years.

Selma Fraiberg wrote a classic book in 1961 on child development, *The Magic Years* that is still popular sixty years later. I heard her speak when she presented at a local university and she had the audience do an exercise that transformed my life. She told us to close our eyes and think of someone we loved. We visualized this person coming into the room and sitting in a chair opposite us and then we told the person why we loved them. I imagined my mother in the opposite chair and told her why I loved her.

Ms. Fraiberg told us to bid this person goodbye and invite ourselves to sit in the opposite chair. She told us to tell ourselves all the reasons we loved ourselves. I could not do it. I struggled and struggled and finally said, "I'm a talented cook." To be comfortable with the truthfulness of this statement I added "but not all the time." I could not go further. After a lengthy pause, I said, "I'm an acceptable parent." Again, I amended this statement with, "but not often enough." I could not think of anything else positive to say, a single quality I could praise without qualifiers. Even though we sat with our eyes closed, I believed everyone around me knew I had nothing positive to say about myself. Many people with ADHD have the ingrained habit of putting themselves down.

Ms. Fraiburg spoke about negative self-talk and the need to be aware of it. Driving home, I decided to give equal rights and equal attention to my thoughts about myself. From that day on I said something positive to counterbalance every negative thought I had about myself. At night, before falling asleep, I reviewed my day and came up with a positive statement for each negative one. With time, all negative self-talk disappeared.

Reading *Learned Optimism, How to Change Your Mind and Your Life* by Martin Seligman provided additional help. This is when I truly learned to eliminate my negativity and replace it with positive thoughts. His simple ideas made a dramatic difference for me. Whenever something went wrong, I talked myself up, not down. I made statements about things within my control that would lead to a better outcome the next time. I may have screwed up this time but that does not mean I screw up all the time. If I didn't do well on a test, I could study harder and get a higher score on the next one.

Whenever I had a problem I pretended it was a fire. What could put out that fire as quickly as possible? What could I say or do to minimize the problem? What could I say or do to move beyond the problem and maintain my self-esteem?

When I was successful at something I took full credit. To use the fire analogy, I made the fire bigger. What could I say to make my success more wonderful and meaningful? What could I say to take as much credit as possible for my success? For example, "I did well because I started on time" or "I got the right people to help" or "I have brilliant ideas."

After recalling everything that contributed to my success, I focused only on my positive thoughts. It amazed me how quickly I stopped the negative self-talk. My new focus on my strengths instead of my weaknesses improved my self-esteem.

Step one, of course, is to realize our negative self-talk. Dr. Amen calls them ANTs—Automatic Negative Thoughts. John, a participant in our support group, said, "I work for the worst boss anyone can imagine. He criticizes me no matter what I do and I can never please him." Then he added, "I'm self-employed."

There is a technique that helps people notice their negative self-talk and stop it. Put a rubber band on your wrist and whenever you say something negative about yourself, snap it. After John had worn the rubber band for several days I asked him how it was going. He replied, "I have a sore wrist!"

Perhaps some people say I was successful before my diagnosis but to me my earlier successes were hit-and-miss and did not build on one another. Now my successes multiply because I can count on them.

Gaining high self-esteem is a sequential process. With each improvement I increased my confidence and capabilities. I take a step, recognize my improvement, and praise myself for my progress. My self-confidence increased as a result. I was improving my life after my diagnosis. Each step takes me slowly towards satisfactory functioning and higher self-esteem.

Self-esteem should not be confused with self-confidence. Self-confidence is recognizing your competence and self-esteem is believing in your worthiness. We build self-esteem the old-fashioned way; we earn it—through dedication, effort and sacrifice. When we have developed self-esteem, we feel whole and satisfied. We show our gratitude by giving generously back to the world, being gracious in victory and graceful in defeat. Self-esteem is crucial to how much or how little contentment we have at the end of our lives.

I read that Angela Madsen, a Paralympian, died at age 60 while rowing from Los Angeles to Honolulu. I looked up the book she wrote, *Rowing Against the Wind.* One of the reviewer's comments on Angela's book perfectly captures how I want to inspire people with ADHD: "[We] should not listen to what others say about us. We need to look inside and see what we are made of and go for it."

ADHD is not a behavior disorder, a mental illness, or a specific learning disability; it is a developmental impairment of the brain's self-management system. It is a neurological disorder that impacts the parts of the brain that help people plan, focus on, and execute tasks.

CHAPTER SIXTEEN

Finding the Humor in ADHD

BEFORE MY DIAGNOSIS I WAS playful and fun. When I was diagnosed I felt there was nothing fun or funny about it. Being cheerful while having ADHD and laughing at the stupid things I did never entered my mind. My self-consciousness about my diagnosis caused me to be inhibited and restrained. Mostly I was ashamed and felt like the scarlet letters ADHD were printed on my forehead. Everyone could see these letters and knew I was damaged goods. I told myself, again and again, "Nothing is different, only now I have a name for it." After I became public about my ADHD I slowly became comfortable having it and even learned that it can be funny.

I once took part in a guided visualization where I gave my future self advice to put more fun back in my life and not to take things so seriously. We then visualized our future selves giving us a gift. As a reminder to lighten up, mine gave me a box of crackerjacks. Now I plan to buy a box of crackerjacks and put the fun back into my life.

People with ADHD do many stupid things but with the proper perspective, our stupid behaviors are hilarious. Around non-ADHD people we hide our ridiculous selves, but with one another, we compete on how stupid we have been.

There used to be a website, *You Know You Have ADHD When...*, where we submitted our most foolish stories. Humor is healthy and we need to laugh at ourselves. When we can laugh at ourselves we have developed a healthy perspective on our lives and our ADHD.

One woman wrote that her brother and sister live with ADHD and she did not think we should joke about it. People responded to her comment by saying that humor helped them realize others have the same struggles and issues. One woman said she was crying and laughing and could not stop reading. Another person said he laughed so hard while reading the website that he shut the windows so his neighbors would not hear him.

Here are several examples from the website, thankfully not all from my life:

- You thought you had lost your eyeglasses until you found them sitting on your head.

- You find the remote control for the DVD player in the refrigerator.

- You search for your watch and then notice it on your wrist.

- You enter a room, do several useful things, come out, sit down and then remember why you went into that room.

- You dial a number but when someone answers, you forget who you called and why.

- Your spouse asks you for a cup of coffee. You walk into the kitchen, forget why you are there and make yourself a peanut butter sandwich.

- You borrow your husband's car keys because you can't find yours. You put his keys on the car roof while you get in. You see your keys on the car seat, use them to start the car, and drive off, wondering what "sounded like keys hitting the pavement."

- Your daughter calls from church and asks why both her mom and dad left in separate cars without her.

- You are halfway to work when you remember you changed jobs two months ago and the new job is in the opposite direction.

- You cut a presentation short to run home because you do not remember turning the lawn sprinkler off. Once home you discover you forgot to turn it on.

- You keep telling people you live in the Alpine Terrace Apartments although you moved from there two years ago. Those apartments were in California and you now live in Georgia.

- You leave to pick your child up at his friend's house and drive right by. You turn around and arrive home . . . without your child.

- Whenever the smoke alarm goes off the comic in your household yells, "It's done."

One of my favorite stories is about a friend who rode his bike home from work for lunch and left it in the driveway. After lunch he got in his car to return to work and ran over his bike.

How often did Steve and I drive our car into our garage with our bikes on the roof rack? When bikes, skis or camping equipment were on top of the car, we learned to hang a tennis ball on a string so that it would dangle in front of the windshield to remind us on our return, "No further or you'll be sorry!"

I once won the Humorous Speech Contest in the local Toastmaster's Club. Everyone roared with laughter as I described my ADHD life. A First-Class Forgetter! Do you remember the joke, "When God passed out ears, I thought He said beers so I asked for two huge frosty ones"? When God passed out brains I thought He said "drains," so I asked for a huge one that emptied quickly."

When I was a child having a terrible memory was troublesome. Can you imagine how annoyed my mother was to ask me for the tenth time to clean up my room? I meant to but I kept forgetting. When I attended graduate school to train as a social worker I learned "reframing." How we talk about something has a lasting impact on us. After I knew about my ADHD and understood how it contributes to my horrendous memory I "reframed."

No longer was I someone with an awful memory. I was someone outstanding at forgetting! I taught my children to do their best at whatever they attempted so I wanted to be the best forgetter ever! I attended five national conferences for adults with ADHD and there's tough competition for the title of "First-Class Forgetter." Still, without false modesty, I am in the top one hundred.

Here are a few examples of my forgetting skills:

First, cars. Everyone with ADHD has a car story. Buying gas and leaving the gas cap behind or driving off after paying for the gas but not pumping it. How many of you drove off while the nozzle was still in the tank pumping gas?

Once when I paid for the gas but did not pump it. I drove home, less than a mile away, and noticed the fuel gauge registered empty. I thought, "The gauge must be broken because I just filled the tank." I drove back to the station to get the gauge repaired. Joe, the station attendant, said,

"I wondered when you would return for the gas you purchased." Then he added, "Here's the credit card you left behind."

How many of you have car key stories? You can't find them when you need them. You do not remember when you last had them. I trained myself to keep my keys in my purse when not in the ignition. I asked Steve and my sons never to take my keys. As a result losing car keys poses little problem for me. Oh sure, there's the "occasional" time of having them when shopping and misplacing them. Don't we all do that?

I never locked my keys in the car because I had to use a key to lock the car. When we purchased a new Honda, the sales associate showed me how to lock the car door without the key. Unhelpful advice! Since then I have locked my keys in the car three times. When we bought the new Honda, thank God, we joined AAA. They come and unlock cars for free.

One summer my friend Mary visited from Australia. We wandered around Seattle's Pike Place Market. After browsing for a few hours I returned to the car to put additional coins in the meter and heard a humming noise. Mary said, "Your car's motor is on." Sure enough. The keys were in the ignition, the car was on and the doors were locked. I called AAA, told them where the car was and enjoyed lunch at a nearby French restaurant. (You would be surprised, and maybe pleased, to learn the yellow pages lists many companies that unlock car doors.)

After unlocking the car and turning the motor off the repairperson delivered the keys to me in the restaurant. Then Mary and I shopped and browsed again. When we returned to the car I could not find my keys. Where had I left them? In which of the many places we visited since lunch? Did we have to retrace all our steps? We started at the restaurant and my lucky day!

Losing one's car requires more skill than losing the keys but I am up to the challenge. I park in the same location every time to save time hunting for a lost car on my weekly shopping trips. If I have to park elsewhere in the lot I tell the attendant at checkout, "No thanks. I can carry the groceries to my car." I don't want company while searching for it.

When I shop at Costco there is no attendant to take my purchases to the car but the lot is bigger and I buy more items. Everything is fine when I leave the store but my carefree attitude vanishes after going down one row of cars and coming up the next. Where is my bleepity-bleeping car? I am sure I parked it in this row! By now, people are staring at me, wondering why I am returning a cartful of items I just purchased.

While vacationing in Florida many years ago I parked a white rental car in a mall parking lot and ran a few errands. When I returned 30 minutes later, my key did not open any of the four white cars in the same area where I had parked mine. My immediate, panicked thought was, "The car's been stolen!"

I called over a mall security guard. He walked to his unmarked white car (which earlier I tried to open) to get the paperwork. While he was gone I realized the only thing I knew about the stolen car was its color. I didn't remember the make, the model or the year; I didn't know the license number or where I rented it. The police report would be, "White car stolen from a parking lot."

When the security guard returned I told him I had changed my mind and no longer wanted to report the car stolen. With a shrug of his shoulders and a loud sigh, he left. Then I feverishly peered inside every white car in the lot. Ten minutes later, hot, sweaty and anxious, I found the little beauty three rows away. With an enormous smile, I got in, rolled down the window, turned up the music and sped off.

Most of you, much younger than I, have had less time to become first-class forgetters. Do not be discouraged. Continue to work on your forgetting skills. Soon you will have enough funny stories to last a lifetime. And remember: reframe. Always reframe!

Myth: Children with ADHD eventually outgrow their disorder.

Fact: Rather than ADHD symptoms getting better as a person reaches adulthood, they can get worse, and it can be the first time that the symptoms are recognized as a problem. ADHD is a 'lifespan disorder' – although symptoms may reduce or increase across the decades.

CHAPTER SEVENTEEN

Honoring My ADHD Positives

I ONCE TOOK PART IN a discussion at a national ADHD conference on the subject, "Can ADHD ever be positive?" It was sparked by Dr. Hallowell's belief that ADHD, if properly managed, is positive.

Is there anything positive about having this disorder, even when properly managed? Or does getting our ADHD "properly managed" make our tough lives less difficult but not exactly positive?

The often-cited positive attributes of ADHD are risk-taking, novelty-seeking, creativity, empathy and curiosity. Are these characteristics truly a part of ADHD in the same way disorganization, procrastination, impulsivity and distractibility are? There is doubt about this. According to Sam Goldstein, Ph.D., no research shows consistent positive traits among people with ADHD.

I am reminded of Louis Braille, blind from birth, who, when asked if he wanted to have sight, answered, "I would prefer more sensitive fingers." He did not understand what the other choice—sightedness—would be like. He believed his life would be easier to navigate if he had fingers that were more sensitive. Likewise, some entrepreneurs—some quite successful—value their ADHD, saying they would not want to be without it. However, even these individuals will admit their ADHD is not a total gift: Glenn Beck, a conservative radio host, has said his ADHD is a gift for his work, but not for his marriage. Despite their successes in life, Ty Pennington and Michael Phelps have been arrested for drunk driving.

I believe most who view their ADHD as a gift fall into the hyperactive/impulsive presentation of ADHD. The high energy aspect of the disorder helps provide them with creative, out-of-the-box ideas, fueling their pre-existing drive to be successful innovators. However, for those of us with inattentive ADHD, it is another story.

Dr. Hallowell writes about "unwrapping the gifts" of ADHD. For me this conjures up the image of a beautiful woman on Christmas morning slowly opening her presents to marvel at her gifts . . . but unwrapping the gifts of ADHD is not like that. It's like receiving a stack of Russian dolls, where removing one only reveals another, then another, and another, until you finally find the tiniest treasure deep inside.

Rather than unwrapping a gift, I think finding the positive aspects of ADHD is like jumping over a series of hurdles before claiming your prize. Here are some of the hurdles:

- Parents or teachers who did not recognize our ADHD during our childhood.

- A widespread belief that ADHD only exists in hyperactive little boys.

- Stigma about ADHD and people not believing it is an actual medical disorder.

- People who minimize the challenges of ADHD by saying, "Everyone has a little bit of ADHD."

- Physicians and therapists who believe you can't have ADHD if you did well in school or who only see depression or anxiety and not your ADHD.

- Problems with procrastination, disorganization, distractibility, forgetfulness, time blindness, low self-esteem, masking, rejection sensitivity and many more.

Those of us with ADHD will never experience life without it. Perhaps, like Mr. Braille's sensitive fingers, our disability gives us special abilities but we will never know if these abilities make up for what we lack.

The question for me is not whether ADHD is a blessing or a curse. My question is, "Am I making the most of what I have and who I am?"

There is no doubt that many people overcome their challenges with ADHD and thrive, but even Dr. Hallowell, who says there are positives to having ADHD, modifies this by saying, "if well-managed." We progress if we work to develop the positive aspects of this disorder.

It reminds me of the phrase, "What we focus on grows." If we focus on the negatives, they will grow. If we focus on the positives, they will expand. It is our choice.

Lisa Poast, my first friend with ADHD, wrote about her experience with ADHD for a newsletter we sent to members of ADD Resources. This is a shortened version.

As I journeyed from a negative to a more positive view of
ADHD, I enjoyed the moments when I recognized and praised
myself for new behaviors, minor accomplishments and completed

tasks. I recall where I started and acknowledge how far I have come. My journey has been difficult (and often I wanted to quit), but I made progress toward my destination. I am on the right road, traveling in the right direction. Positive thoughts nourish me so I keep traveling.

I learned to travel lightly, no longer carrying baggage from my past. I am a seasoned traveler, capable of figuring out how to pass through any rough landscape. I am confident in my abilities and strong in knowing I survived. As my journey gets easier, I even enjoy it. I travel down the open road of life, sometimes skipping, sometimes trudging, and sometimes limping but usually with a song in my heart, a twinkle in my eye and a smile on my face. My journey through life is the adventure I dreamed it would be.

My life improved after my diagnosis but even before my diagnosis, my ADHD drove me to live an interesting and exciting life. I was always willing and eager to take on risks and challenges, especially of a physical nature. I value physical activity. As my body parts wore out or suffered injuries I eliminated several sports I enjoyed. However, I read that rowing was easy on the knees and provided a strenuous workout. After my second total knee replacement, this time to my right knee, I strengthened my body on the rowing machine at the YMCA.

One night I had an inspired thought: "I want to row on the water." I searched the internet for rowing instruction and located the website of

Larry who offered lessons on Commencement Bay, just down the hill from where we live.

Although I had a distressing history with Commencement Bay, my desire to row on the water overrode my residual fears.

Larry's website stated, "Anyone between 12 and 60 can learn to row." I was 74! Would my age be a deal breaker? I emailed him, explained my interest, and mentioned my age. Larry sent a positive response, giving his age as 75! His first lesson was free so potential students could make an informed decision about continuing with the lessons. I took my first lesson in May 2018, when the air and water were brisk. Larry helped me into an open water shell that is more stable than a flatwater shell.

I quickly realized rowing on the water is more complicated than rowing on a machine. More muscles are engaged to keep the scull in balance. There are the oars to manage. I had to place them vertically in the water at the beginning of the stroke and rotate them at the end when taking them out of the water so they were parallel to the water before starting another stroke. I could not let the oars dig too deeply into the water and I could not raise them too high when I brought them out. I had to cross one hand under the other hand so the oar handles did not collide.

There was so much to learn and I was overwhelmed. I rowed down the waterway with Larry, close by in his scull, giving me instructions.

On the way back, when the lesson was over, I had to move out of the way of a boat cruising by. The boat's wake pushed my scull toward a boat moored at a nearby dock. Larry shouted, "Don't let the oar get behind you." What did he mean by that? I soon found out. The scull capsized and I was pitched into the water. I could not climb back into the overturned scull but I was not worried. Even fully clothed with my shoes on I could swim to the nearby dock. That is when I learned the dock was two feet above me and I could not hoist myself out of the water.

Now I worried. So near and yet so far and I was getting cold. Larry solved the problem. He rowed forward so the front end of his scull went under the dock. This maneuver stabilized his scull. I crawled onto the scull's deck and sat there while he rowed us back to shore. That was my introduction to rowing on Commencement Bay.

I didn't tell Steve about my inauspicious beginning. I intended to return for additional lessons and I didn't want him to talk me out of it as we both remembered my near death in Commencement Bay years earlier.

Initially I was anxious whenever waves rocked my scull. Would I fall in the water again? With practice I learned to rest the oar blades on the water to stabilize the scull and overcame my fear of capsizing. But I never developed the confidence to be on the water by myself and recognized that I never would.

Rowing is a perfect activity for someone with ADHD. It engages the body and the mind, requiring us to focus on executing each stroke with proper form. Whether inside on a rowing machine or outside on Commencement Bay, rowing is now my favorite physical activity, a challenge I have fully embraced.

Dr. Rakesh Jain, a psychiatrist, believes one symptom of ADHD that should be included in the DSM-5 but is not is how often we will not attempt something because we fear failure. Our history of past failures stops us from trying again. Brendan Mahan, an ADHD Coach, calls this "Our Wall of Awful."

I knew Bruce had a Wall of Awful. When he was a child he would not try anything new unless he was sure of success, but I didn't have a Wall of Awful. I am not afraid to try things. Nevertheless, the longer I thought about it, I realized I, too, had a Wall of Awful.

Graduating from Wheaton College required a certain proficiency in a foreign language. I didn't pass the language proficiency test and had to take a year of beginning German at college despite taking two years of German in high school! I told myself, "I can't learn a foreign language." I didn't try to learn the local language in Malawi with the Peace Corps. When vacationing in Mexico I didn't know more than "por favor" and "gracias." It felt disrespectful not to attempt more but believing "I cannot learn a foreign language." held me back.

As a child I took piano lessons for three years but never progressed. No one would ever want to hear me play. "I can't play a musical instrument" was added to my Wall of Awful.

After my ADHD diagnosis I heard a clinician say, "People with ADHD can learn anything. They just have to learn the way that works for them." I bought a classical guitar and took lessons for over a year, trying to learn in a way that worked for me. But I never found it and sadly concluded again, "I cannot play a musical instrument."

When I was ten years old I tried out for our church choir. My sister Melissa was a choir member and I attended a practice with her. I sang the first hymn when the choirmaster abruptly stopped us and called out, "Who is the monotone?" I was the only new person. I was the monotone so I told myself, "I can't sing."

Whenever I pondered what I wanted changed in my life if reborn (how often do we ask ourselves this question?), I wanted to play an instrument or sing. When I told Larry, my rowing coach, "I can't sing. I'm a monotone," he replied, "My wife teaches singing and claims she can teach anyone." His response made me wonder if I were not a hopeless case. I signed up for weekly singing lessons.

It took a year of lessons for me to match pitches. For the uninitiated this is step one for singers—hear a tone and match it with your voice. This is what orchestra members do when the first violin gives them a tone. They check their instruments are tuned to match the violin's tone. Children have a natural ability to match tones if they are encouraged in their singing. If not encouraged or, as in my case, discouraged, the ability fades away and it is a long, slow road to recovery.

I had no goals for my singing lessons until I heard about the Tacoma Refugee Choir. It meets weekly at the church I attend although it is not affiliated with the church. I participated in one of the choir's public sing-a-longs and had fun, then joined the non-auditioned choir and attended its weekly practices. I shocked my singing teacher when I told her, "I joined the Tacoma Refugee Choir." I imagine she thought I was not ready for public performance.

The choir members are refugees and people who warmly welcome refugees. Although I am the oldest, it has people of all ages, and many have outstanding voices. They step forward to sing solos while the choir joins them to sing the chorus.

I have sung in two public concerts, one at a local university where students and community members watched and later joined us in singing, and the other in a Christmas program with the Tacoma Symphony. The songs we sing are emotional, about refugees wanting homes, to be safe and to be valued. A student made a video of our program and watching it on the choir's website brings tears to my eyes.

Myth: ADHD is something created by pharmaceutical company to increase their profits.
Fact: If you go back a century in medical literature you read descriptions of children who sound as though they have ADHD. It is a condition found throughout the world in children and adults.

CHAPTER EIGHTEEN

My ADHD Activism

IN 1993, THE YEAR after my diagnosis, I attended the first conference in the US for adults with ADHD held at the University of Michigan in Ann Arbor. While reading a book on the shuttle bus from the airport to the university, a man named Tom, whom I didn't know, repeatedly tried to converse with me. (Given that he was interrupting a stranger reading on a bus, I should have realized sooner that Tom had ADHD and was going to the same conference!)

It turned out that Tom was from Tacoma, and a few months after the conference, we started a support group in our hometown for adults with ADHD, using space provided free by a local hospital. Of course, we did not know how to run such a group and faced many challenges.

Our first challenge was keeping the participants on topic. People with ADHD have a hard time with that and veer off on tangents they consider relevant but their listeners find irrelevant. We lack filters and it is hard for us to focus. We need to start at the beginning and share the entire history of something instead of focusing on the immediate situation. We see the big picture but often get lost in irrelevancies.

As the group leader I wanted to be polite and encourage participants to talk freely. They would not return if they did not find the meeting helpful. Yet I became fidgety and irritable when I didn't have the skill to keep the speakers on track.

Besides meandering talkers, a few participants talked on and on. I could not restrain myself and cried out, "You've talked long enough!" Carol, one of the talkative ones, took offense. She came to the next meeting armed with a stopwatch to time everyone who talked. She commented after each speaker, "I didn't talk as long as that."

Our support group had additional problems. Each month new people came and each new arrival had to tell her or his life story. This left no time for the returning participants to share what was happening in their lives. Many people arrived late. Because the group members varied each month, participants did not get to know one another well enough to establish trust and be open about their situations. A last concern was the range of challenges the participants faced. Some were financially well off, while others were on food stamps and Medicaid. A few had done well in life while others were living borderline lives. We could not find common ground to discuss the group's needs and problems.

Yet sometimes we did find common ground as we all had ADHD. A 21-year-old man named Sam touched us with a story about how life can quickly go south. One day, late for work, a cop stopped him for speeding. Sam's vehicle registration had expired. He got a speeding ticket, his license was suspended and he was ordered to appear in court with a valid registration. Sam kept driving with a suspended license (he could not pay for the new registration and the ticket unless he continued to work), was stopped again by the police and got a larger fine. Sam forgot his court date and lost his job for being late too often.

We all related to his story. We understood how our minor issues become big ones because of distraction, running late, procrastinating or forgetting. If only Sam left for work on time. If only he renewed his registration when it was due. If only he remembered his court date. We fill our lives with regrets and "if only's."

Because of the numerous challenges we faced, our support group disbanded. I tried to think of another way to help adults with ADHD and switched to a different format—a monthly speaker with information helpful to people with ADHD followed by a Q & A. Another hospital gave us free use of its auditorium one evening a month. The meetings were held for 15 years with 30–40 attendees each month.

The new format worked better but not perfectly. People sometimes interrupted the speaker with their questions. Some presenters were more skilled than others at managing the audience. During the Q&A several participants took a long time explaining their situations before asking their question.

I created a schedule for the upcoming six months and promoted the meetings by bringing fliers to the offices of pediatricians and psychiatrists.

I needed to prepare myself emotionally for the group's initial meeting because I would "out" myself publicly for the first time as someone with ADHD. The previous support group was small, with only five or six people, and it was confidential. I had an ADHD friend there so I didn't feel alone. This meeting was different. It would be a much larger public meeting and not all attendees might have ADHD. I felt more exposed and vulnerable, mainly because I was visibly in charge. I felt the pressure to model healthy ADHD behavior, announcing I have the condition without making it a huge deal.

How could I announce, "I have ADHD" when I was ashamed to have it?

Fortunately I had a role model who dealt with his ADHD in a healthy way, a man who openly told one and all, "I have ADHD" without feeling diminished by saying it—Dr. Edward Hallowell. A presenter at the conference in Michigan, Dr. Hallowell was a graduate of Harvard and Tulane Medical School. He self-diagnosed his ADHD after hearing a professor lecture about the condition in children. He told me he was never reluctant to say, "I have ADHD" because he never believed it was anything to be ashamed of. I wanted to get to the same stage of mental health, able to tell anyone without anxiety or shame.

To prepare for the meeting I visualized saying to a packed auditorium, "My name is Cynthia Hammer and I have ADHD." Practicing this wording aloud made my stomach queasy and my mouth dry. My voice quavered as I spoke and that was unacceptable. I sat in the privacy of my car and said my introductory piece, repeatedly, until I could say, without apprehension, without fear, "I am Cynthia Hammer and I have ADHD."

Still I was unsure if I was ready to go public. I was committed to being open and honest, but I remained scared. What if someone who knew me was at the meeting? Would the audience accept me after it learned I have ADHD? Would people wonder about the quality of the presentation if someone with ADHD organized it?

At our first meeting, instead of the hundred attendees I visualized, 35 people sat in the audience. Announcing I have ADHD was easy. After my first public disclosure, it became easier and easier for me to tell others. I learned that most people quickly forget because it is not as important to them as I worried it would be.

With time and the new life Dr. Smith predicted for me, having ADHD became less important to me as well. I even became comfortable talking to community groups about ADHD.

Once when speaking to a Rotary group at a luncheon, I used a meta-phor about eating to help them understand the life experiences of living as an adult with ADHD. I told them the following story:

Suzie Smith was born with one hand tied behind her back. No one, not her parents, her friends, or even her teachers noticed this. Even Suzie did not realize there was something different about her. Suzie was remarkably dainty whenever the school cafeteria served soup, never slurping, never spilling. When she left the table as neat as she found it, others commented, "What a sweet, lovely girl. So proper and well-mannered!"

On other days the school cafeteria served meat. Suzie needed two hands to cut it into bite-sized pieces. She did poorly on these days. It took her a long time to eat and often she did not finish. She was messy, leaving scraps and drippings on the table and floor. People were surprised and thought she was messy on purpose.

They would say, "What's wrong with you? Why are you messy today? If you tried harder, you would be successful." Suzie endured her childhood hearing disparaging comments almost daily.

Then one day, when she was 35, she was eating fish tacos in a fancy restaurant. The server blurts out, "Why are you eating with one hand tied behind your back?"

Imagine Suzie's surprise and relief as she understands why she struggled all those years. Imagine her despair as she compre-hends how different her life would have been if only someone had noticed her hand tied behind her back sooner. However, just by knowing she has this limitation, Suzie stops being so hard on herself. She understands there are others in her situation whose lives are as constrained as hers.

Suzie wants to find out what it's like to be two-handed but untying her hand is a complex process. Few doctors learned in their training that people have this condition. Even doctors knowledgeable about her situation are still trying to figure out the best way to free her hand. What medication? In what dose? Will it even help?

Suzie is fortunate: her doctor, after several false attempts, frees her hand with the right medication. Yet no amount of treatment or therapy will make her released hand function perfectly. Diagnosis and treatment freed the hand tied behind Suzie's back, but that is all it does. That is all it can do.

What Suzie does with her hand once freed is up to her. If Suzie wants her released hand to be useful, it will take motivation and work. Medication is only part of the treatment; "pills don't teach skills," as they say. Any improvement after medication is up to Suzie. She must strengthen the muscles in her hand that have been unused since birth. She has to learn and practice coping skills and acquire new habits.

Some people deny that they have one hand tied behind their backs. They deny that having only one good hand causes problems. Some even believe being one-handed gives them special abilities. They worry that if they untie their hand, they will lose their inclination toward risk-taking, novelty-seeking, creativity, empathy, and love of learning. They decide not to have their hand untied.

I did not like having one-hand tied behind my back. Sure, it gave me a few special abilities but also several disabilities. I wanted to reduce my disabilities and maintain my special abilities. So far, it is working.

Although Suzie's story is not directly about me living with undiagnosed ADHD for 49 years, I never tell the story without getting emotional. My hurt feelings come flooding back and my voice quivers. People in the audience with this disorder also get emotional. They share their experiences of living with an unrecognized disability and recall the times others made belittling and negative comments about how they performed. They understand the costs of living with just one hand.

I would tell them that "recovering" from ADHD is like climbing a circular staircase. Each improved habit we adopt, like putting the credit card back where it belongs or getting to appointments on time, moves us another step up the circular staircase. Each step up enhances our lives, increases our control and strengthens our self-esteem.

I n 1994, two years after starting the ADHD Support group, I founded and headed the non-profit organization ADD Resources, to help adults learn about ADHD. My position allowed me to use all the positives—risk-taking, novelty-seeking, empathy, creativity, and love of learning—and challenged me to keep the negatives at bay.

My experience as co-president of the League of Women Voters gave me the confidence to start ADD Resources that I led for 15 years. Many organizations hire an attorney to create a non-profit but I did not. I read the requirements, completed the application and the IRS approved our organization to be a non-profit, a 501(c) 3. I continued to be reluctant to hire "experts" when I could learn to run a non-profit on my own, not by getting a degree in Non-Profit Management. I created our website after a friend taught me the basics. I managed the organization's finances by learning to use QuickBooks.

An ADHD positive that I have always valued is my need to undertake interesting activities, not to be bored, and not to be stuck in a rut. The challenges I faced and the expertise required made growing ADD Resources interesting and exciting. Because I was starting a new organization I used my creativity every day.

At first ADD Resources existed at my desk in our home's basement. When I started the organization all three sons lived at home. After they moved out, I converted one bedroom into my home office. I was unpaid, although after being the director for ten years, I received a salary of $1,000 monthly for unlimited work hours.

Working for ADD Resources was my labor of love, my joy. Within a few years we hired a part-time secretary and then committed to renting office space. After a few more years, we rented a larger office space. My risk-taking was at work when we assumed expenses without knowing how to pay for them. The same risk-taking excitement was at work when we invited national authorities to present at our conferences, never sure the conference receipts would cover their fees.

One of my ideas was to compile articles written by adults with ADHD and the professionals who diagnose and treat us to produce a 125-page booklet called *The ADD Reader*. It was popular because adults with limited attention preferred reading short articles containing concise information. *The Reader* was only available to members of ADD

Resources. Membership also gave them a discount at our conferences and allowed them to borrow books, videotapes, and audiotapes from our lending library. Our membership grew to over 800 adults with ADHD.

Before we hosted our first conference, I scoured the area for a centrally located facility with a reasonable rental fee and free parking. Foster High School in Renton met all the criteria and for many years we held our conferences and workshops there. We used the cafeteria for book sales and food service, the classrooms for breakout sessions and the main auditorium for keynote addresses.

As our organization became widely known, the phone rang every day with people calling for advice about their concerns. At first, I enjoyed answering the callers' questions but over time, I didn't want to hear any more life stories. My empathy for adults with ADHD was better expressed through managing the organization's activities. I was relieved when our secretary, Joan Jager, had a remarkable ability to talk with the people who called for support and advice.

I was the Director of ADD Resources for 15 years and grew it to national prominence. I hired staff, learned bookkeeping, organized monthly public meetings, and wrote and published a monthly newsletter. We sponsored an annual conference with national authorities as presenters and over 300 attendees, including adults with ADHD and the professionals who help them. We provided workshops for teachers to educate them about ADHD and how to help the children in their classrooms with this diagnosis.

I could not have created this organization before my diagnosis and treatment. Dr. Smith was right—I have a new life.

A reporter interviewed me about ADHD for our local newspaper and asked, "What has changed since your diagnosis?" I had little to tell her, maybe because my diagnosis was thirteen years earlier and the improvements were subtle, gradual and seemingly insignificant. But what a difference they made—having my clothes in order, knowing where

I put my keys and credit card, creating and sticking to a list, completing even tedious tasks, remembering things I needed to do (still a challenge), being aware when I was interrupting or tuning out and starting and finishing tasks on time.

It may have embarrassed me to tell the reporter of these seemingly minor achievements. They sounded trivial, simple and easily achieved by most people. I finally told her "Before my diagnosis I never could have established and become the Executive Director of a non-profit organization called ADD Resources. I could never have made this non-profit prosper and become a national organization that helped thousands of adults with this disorder learn about their condition and how to improve their lives."

My answer impressed her and helped her understand how different my life had become.

I thrived as Director of ADD Resources. Even though I continued to have challenges, I recognized my strengths—having creative ideas, organizing successful events and motivating volunteers. I stayed calm and confident, helpful when putting on events as they always have stressful moments. I learned not to worry and to go with the flow.

Sometimes I had unrealistic expectations for our conferences, visualizing 500 or more people attending. When that was not to be, I made a mental switch and focused on hosting the best conference regardless of attendance. Steve helped by telling me, "ADD Resources is a non-profit. Your focus should be on helping people, not on making money."

Adults with ADHD perform well in crisis because we hyperfocus and zero in on the important things that need to be done. Two episodes come to mind where I dealt with potential crises at our conferences.

First, the keynote speaker for one of our annual conferences, Dr. Peter Jensen, a psychiatrist on the staff of Columbia University, was coming from New York City. Although I called his office several times for information on his travel plans, I had not heard from him. Dr. Jensen had not told me where he was staying and whether we needed to pick him up. By 8:30 am, he still had not arrived and he was to present at 9 am.

Quickly shifting gears, I approached a local physician attending the conference. "Dr. Mandelkorn, can you be our keynote speaker if Dr. Jensen doesn't arrive in time?" He said, "I'm glad to fill in. Let's see if he gets here."

In typical ADHD fashion (for he, too, has this diagnosis), Dr. Peter Jensen strolled in at 8:40 am, splendidly dressed in a pink and black pinstriped shirt and a darker pink bow tie.

"I'm so glad to see you," I said, presenting as calm an exterior as possible. Then, sounding slightly annoyed, I asked, "Where have you been?"

He replied, "I have family that lives in the area and was visiting with them. Are we set to go?"

For another conference our work crew arrived two hours early to set up for book sales, registration and coffee service. When we arrived the janitor said, "All the electricity is off in the building. There's been a major power outage in the neighborhood and we haven't learned when it will be restored." After a few moments while we digested the information the janitor returned and said, "The junior high, just a block away, has power and I got permission for your conference to relocate there."

I said to the volunteer crew, "Okay gang! Let's get to work. Two of you help the janitor hang a sheet in the gym for a screen and set up chairs for 250 people. Joan and Judy, take care of registration. The rest of you help Nancy set up the food and Deborah set up the bookstore. We'll work out where the breakout sessions will be during the keynote presentation."

Everyone hustled and we started the conference in the new location just 15 minutes late. We managed extremely well in this emergency.

As Director of ADD Resources I continued to make verbal commitments to ensure my follow through. By telling one or two friends what I planned to do, I made sure I did it. I learned not to promise more than I could deliver. Having gigantic ideas is inspiring but if we have a profusion of ideas that go unrealized, people lose confidence in our organization.

My ADHD challenges have never disappeared but have become less burdensome over the years. My improved self-talk that I have practiced since I heard Selma Fraiburg's presentation, my optimistic approach to life, thanks to Dr. Seligman, my medication and my efforts to improve my performance have all helped me be successful. Serving as the Director of ADD Resources made me competent and confident. I used my strengths and developed new skills and abilities. It, so far, has been the most rewarding 15 years of my life.

However, after 15 many years, the work became repetitive. Because I lacked fresh ideas and inspiration, I resigned and found a new challenge: serving as an ADHD coach. During my coach training I was surprised to learn it required an entirely new body of knowledge and skills, very different from what I learned as a social worker. Instead of focusing on emotions and insights, I helped clients focus on problems, strategies and goals. As a coach, I was more active and talkative in the helping process, analyzing challenges and assisting the client institute lasting changes. It was satisfying to observe the growth in my clients and I enjoyed coaching for several years until I finally retired.

Myth: Children who take ADHD medications will become drug abusers.*

Fact: Research demonstrates that children who take their ADHD medication as prescribed into adolescence have no increased drug usage than teenagers without ADHD. Treating ADHD with medication reduces the likelihood that a child with ADHD will abuse substances. These findings make intuitive sense as ADHD medications reduce the symptoms of the disorder that lead to illicit drug use.

https://www.adhdevidence.org/blog/myths-about-the-treatment-of-adhd

CHAPTER NINETEEN

Marriage and ADHD

THE PERSON ONE MARRIES makes an enormous difference, especially when ADHD is present. I am fortunate that Steve is my husband. He is thoughtful, does not make quick decisions and takes his time when choices need to be made. Sometimes I am impatient with his deliberative approach but he has frequently saved me from an impulsive and faulty decision. He encourages me to pursue my interests. Writing this memoir made me realize how accepting of me Steve has been. He never shamed me for being his high-maintenance, costly wife.

It is sweet that he never thought there was anything "wrong" with me. He accepted me as I was and only occasionally grumbled, "Are you still taking that medication?" implying I did not need it. Now that he is retired, he wonders if he was too caught up in his life to notice what was happening in mine. However, he watched out for me. When Bruce's friend, Tan, got engaged, he told us, "I want to be like Dr. Hammer. I want to care for my wife like he takes care of you."

I thought of most of the things we did but he was my willing partner. Correction: he suggested we go to Malawi with the Peace Corps and years later, he suggested we visit China. But I suggested sailing the San Juan Islands, hiking around Mont Blanc, biking in Japan and biking across the United States. He was my always-willing companion!

Shortly after my diagnosis I asked Steve, "What do you believe is my greatest strength and weakness?" He replied, "Compassion and obliviousness." This sounded contradictory. How can I be compassionate if I am oblivious?

Here is how I explained it to myself.

Oblivious means I am in my own world. I have thoughts unconnected to what others discuss. If I join the conversation, what I contribute is off-kilter because I was not fully tuned in. Sometimes I bump into people or spill things because I don't pay attention to where I am or where others are. Occasionally, because I am direct, I say something that offends or hurts another person's feelings. I am unaware of the impact my words have on the other person. However, if I notice another person's pain, I am compassionate and caring.

When I was diagnosed I said, "It's not like I'm diagnosed with cancer or MS where the probability is I will get worse. With an ADHD diagnosis my life will only improve." And it has. However, my focus was on how I improved. I was unaware of how my relationship with my husband improved until last week when I had an "ah-ha" moment.

I took part in an ADHD Skill Building Telecourse. For an assignment we were to ask another person what he thought were our most salient characteristics. When I asked Steve, he said "creative" and "considerate." I almost fell off my chair in shock! For several years Steve said, "You never consider me. I feel like I always come in last." I tried to be considerate all those years but he did not get the message. I don't know what I am doing differently but to him I am different. He says I am considerate!

Someone with ADHD asked me for advice before marrying another person with ADHD. I should clarify that Steve was never diagnosed with ADHD although he has a few traits. I based my advice on what we learned in our marriage and on my broader knowledge of ADHD.

Both people must be diagnosed and treated for their ADHD. They need a thorough understanding of the condition and how it affects their lives. They need to value and accept themselves as people with many talents who also have ADHD. They should manage their separate lives reasonably well and not expect their marriage partner to fill in any gaps in their performance. They must be tolerant and patient with one another (not common attributes in people with ADHD). For example, I ask Steve to check the dates on the theater tickets but he keeps forgetting. By the time he checks, the play has left town. I don't get upset or say something nasty because I do many things that annoy him and he does not harp on them with me.

In our marriage we give each other space. We do many activities separately and some activities together. When doing something together we help each other. "Did you remember the car keys?" "Did you pack the water purifier?" "What about the sun lotion?" But when he misplaces something, I let him look for it unless it is an urgent need. Then I help him.

Having clear expectations of who does what in managing the household is vital. For example, Steve does most of the yard work but when he is swamped, I help. We assist each other but do not keep track of who is helping whom and how often. It should come out evenly or one marriage partner will become resentful. "I'm always helping you!"

Know the person for an extended time before marrying until the burst of enthusiasm for someone new and different has worn off. Dr.

Amen reports a high infidelity rate among couples where one partner has ADHD. That person seeks novelty and excitement again, only this time outside of the marriage. Couples have a high divorce rate when one or both have ADHD.

When heading into marriage be sure you both strongly value the marital commitment. A couple once told me their psychiatrist was astonished that they had stayed married. The husband has ADHD, the wife has bipolar disorder and their two children have ADHD. Asked how they stayed together, my friend answered, "We both were strongly committed to being married."

What follows is advice for couples where one person has ADHD and the non-ADHD spouse does not believe the condition exists or does not accept their partner's ADHD behaviors. This advice comes from someone who lives on a farm. He compares marriage to a team of workhorses.

> *I don't know how many horses you've been around but, at one time, finding a matched set of horses to pull a wagon was worth more than anything else. With a matched set the ride is smoother and the horses pull longer and farther than an unmatched set. A matched set has a similar gait, one horse leads and the other follows. They aren't fighting each other and pulling unequally. If they pull unequally, they develop sore spots where the harness rubs their flesh. They need to rest more often and are grumpier because they're sore.*
>
> *It's much the same with a husband and wife. If you aren't pulling together, the result could be a living hell.*

His words resonated with me. Over the years Steve and I have learned and learned again maintaining our relationship is more important than the annoyances along the way. We have been married for 51 years and our relationship, like fine wine, has matured.

This past winter Steve drove 90 minutes to cross-country ski for the day. On the ski trail he dropped his car keys and did not realize they were missing until he returned to the car. His cell phone was locked in the car so he borrowed someone's phone to ask me to come and get him. I am almost positive he did not ask me to bring the spare key to his car.

After driving halfway there, I realized I had not brought the spare key but had come too far to turn around. When I arrived, his car was the only one in the lot and he was not there. He appeared 15 minutes later and apologized for keeping me waiting. He had skied the trail again, unsuccessfully searching for his keys. Then I said, "I forgot to bring the key to your car. We have to come back tomorrow." He replied, "Fine."

How can I not love someone who accepts my mistakes without complaint? When I asked him about this he replied, "We've learned to be patient with one another."

ADHD can co-exist, to a greater or less degree, with dyspraxia (difficulty with movement and motor control); dyslexia (difficulty with reading); dysgraphia (difficulty with writing); dyscalculia (difficulty with math); Autism Spectrum Disorder (ASD) and Tourette's.

Time is a Gift

I HAVE LOVED MY MANY unique experiences and memorable adventures. The lows in my life enabled me to appreciate the highs. I don't know, and cannot know, what my life would have been without ADHD but my life has been and continues to be interesting and exciting. I would not trade that for anything.

The movie *Shadowlands* is about the love between a proper, repressed, conservative English professor, C.S. Lewis, and an outgoing, outspoken and sometimes outrageous American divorcee, Joy Davidman. They've been married for four years when Joy learns she is dying of cancer. Although I am a romantic and vicariously experienced the couple's emotional roller coaster, the part of the story that remains with me is Joy's philosophy of life.

Beneath the couple's happiness, there's an undercurrent of sadness. They found happiness only to realize it was time limited. Their joyful times were broken by Joy's winces of pain and sudden fatigue—continual reminders of the fleeting nature of life. Lewis wants to believe Joy is not ill, to focus only on their happy times. Joy maintains that they must acknowledge and accept their sorrow to appreciate their happiness. She believes by knowing one side of life, anguish and pain, they better appreciate and value the other, contentment and joy. If their troubled and unhappy times are unacknowledged, their happy times will be less treasured, their joyful times less valued.

In the movie Lewis and Joy drive to a peak and look down on a valley. Their car trip symbolizes an acceptance of life's entire fabric, the peaks and the valleys. In our culture we seek the "good life"—having sufficient money, memorable experiences, good health, devoted family and friends, and few worries. While no one seeks difficulties or wishes hardship on another, imagine how bland and boring the world would be if we all lived the "good life" and lived it our entire lives.

Perhaps my New England background shows but how would we develop "character?"

I lived the good life until 28 years old. The "tragedies" in my life were not getting my driver's license at 16 and not getting into the college of my choice. When I married Steve I thought my "good life" was secured. He was considerate, honest, handsome and a future surgeon. I was earning my master's degree in social work. It never occurred to me that my life would not always be wonderful, that we would not always be happy.

I look back and wonder how I lived to age 28 with these beliefs intact.

When I was 27 I gave birth to Allison and when I was 28, she died. I learned that no one can count on life being the way we want it to be. After Allison's death Steve said, "I should have put the pills away." He believed he was responsible for her death but I was responsible, not Steve. Repeatedly, I recalled the times I inadequately watched Allison, the times I put her at risk through my inattentiveness. I buried my hurt, pain, and sorrow of her death inside. For 23 years I told only one person, a mother who also had a child die, that I had a baby daughter who died.

I was an unfit mother. How could I have caused my daughter's death? How could I ever care for another child? Twenty-two years after Allison's death I was diagnosed with inattentive ADHD. My diagnosis revived my grief for our daughter, Steve, and me.

Now, years after my diagnosis, I accept it all—the good in my life and the bad. My work to get ADHD in adults recognized and understood helps as I bond with those who struggle to manage their lives in concert with society's expectations.

If your life only contains good fortune, that is your "good fortune." Troubles, problems, sadness and sorrow can come knocking anytime on anyone's door.

On a shelf in our bedroom sits a little, gold-colored cardboard box weighing 1 lb. 12 oz. The white label on the box says:

Bleitz Funeral Home

316 Florentia Street   -   Seattle, Washington
This package contains the cremated remains of

ALLISON MARION HAMMER

Date of death: January 21, 19 73

We lived in Seattle for over a year after Allison's death but we never went for her ashes. We talked about going but never did. We left Seattle for Kentucky. Two years later, we moved to Tacoma, only 30 miles from Seattle, but still we did not go. Many years passed. When I feared the funeral home would dispose of her ashes I called and was told to come. We brought her remains home in the little gold box but that was all we did. It was too hurtful to consider a final parting.

Several times we talked about what we should do. "What about planting a tree in the backyard and putting her ashes beneath it?" I asked, but then answered myself. "No, that won't work. What will happen when we leave this house? I don't want her left behind. I don't want her left with other people."

Then we talked about bringing her when we hiked at Mt. Rainer and releasing her to the wind in one of our favorite places on the mountain. My brothers, sister and I did this with our parents' ashes, releasing them at a lake where they had gone for years after dinner to swim, read their books and enjoy the peaceful setting. They sat in collapsible chairs on a treed hillside that overlooked the lake, often commenting, "Isn't it a glorious evening?"

I was familiar with the drill: carry the ashes to a favorite place, open the container and let the ashes flow with the breeze. However, in researching our plan for Mt. Rainer, we learned it was illegal to dispose of ashes in a national park. Years passed. We thought of going out on a boat in Commencement Bay and spilling the ashes over the side but we never followed through. More years passed.

Finally, when writing our wills, we decided to combine our ashes with Allison's and have them tossed to the winds. She will stay with us until then, in the cardboard box, on a shelf, in our bedroom.

Life is difficult. Accept that and the rest becomes easier. My struggles have enabled me to accept everything in my life. I no longer say, "I live the good life." Instead, I say, "I live a full life. I have experienced the range of life's emotions, from fear to courage, anger to peace and contentment, anxiety to confidence, and depression to happiness. While we cannot always control what happens in our lives, we can control our response and in our responses, we determine the kind of people we are."

I am not an impulsive shopper but when I saw a poster with the words below and a picture of two children fully absorbed in the moment, I bought it. It reminds me to make the most of life. For a life to have meaning and depth, we must accept everything. Each event has meaning and value, even if the meaning and value are only to make us who we are, and to give our journey its unique and special character.

Enjoying.

Paying attention.

No hurry to get on to something

more important.

Whatever we are doing is important,

experiencing each moment

along the way.

Time is a gift.

ADDENDUM

Symptoms of Inattentive ADHD with Examples for Adults

This questionnaire is made available as a public service by the non-profit organization, the Inattentive ADHD Coalition (www.iadhd.org) and was created by Cynthia Hammer, MSW, Executive Director. It is derived from the DSM-5 symptoms of ADHD-Primarily Inattentive and examples of adult inattentive ADHD from the DIVA-2.

Note: *Often* means at least three times a week.

1. I often find it difficult to pay attention to details, or I make careless mistakes in my work.

☐ Makes careless mistakes

☐ Works slowly to avoid mistakes

☐ Works too quickly and therefore makes mistakes

☐ Does not read instructions carefully

☐ Overlooks or misses details

☐ Work is inaccurate

☐ Gets easily bogged down by details

☐ Spends too much time completing detailed tasks

2. I often find it difficult to maintain attention on tasks.

- ☐ Quickly distracted by own thoughts or associations
- ☐ Easily distracted by unrelated thoughts
- ☐ Asks questions about subjects that have already been discussed
- ☐ Difficulty remaining focused during lectures and/or conversations
- ☐ Finds it difficult to watch a film through to the end or to read a book (unless it is something that interests me)
- ☐ Quickly becomes bored with things (unless it is something that interests me)
- ☐ Not able to keep attention on tasks for long (unless it is something that interests me)

3. I often find it challenging to listen even when spoken to directly.

- ☐ Dreamy or preoccupied
- ☐ Difficulty concentrating on a conversation
- ☐ Afterward, not knowing what a conversation was about
- ☐ Usually, I change the subject of a conversation
- ☐ Others say my thoughts are elsewhere
- ☐ My mind seems lost in the clouds, even when there is no obvious distraction

4. I often find it difficult to follow instructions, finish work or complete chores.

☐ Muddles things together and never completes

☐ Starts tasks but quickly loses focus and gets easily sidetracked

☐ Needs a time limit to complete tasks

☐ Difficulty completing administrative tasks

☐ Difficulty following instructions from a manual

5. I often find it challenging to organize tasks and activities.

☐ Difficulty planning activities of daily life

☐ Inflexible because of the need to keep to schedules

☐ Difficulty managing sequential tasks

☐ Can't create an agenda or use a diary or planner consistently

☐ Plans too many tasks or non-efficient planning

☐ Creates schedules but doesn't use them

☐ Regularly books things to take place at the same time (double-booking)

☐ Needs other people to structure things

☐ House and/or workplace are disorganized

☐ Difficulty keeping materials and belongings in order

☐ Work is messy and confusing

☐ Poor sense and management of time

☐ Arrives late

☐ Fails to meet deadlines

6. I often avoid, dislike, or am reluctant to do tasks that require a sustained mental effort (such as reading lengthy instructions or completing my tax return).

☐ Do the easiest or most attractive activities first

☐ Often postpone tedious or difficult tasks

☐ Does not like reading due to mental effort

☐ Avoidance of tasks that require a lot of concentration

☐ Avoids preparing reports, completing forms, or reviewing lengthy papers

☐ Postpone tasks so that deadlines are missed

☐ Avoid monotonous work, such as administration

7. I often lose items needed for tasks and activities.

☐ Mislays tools, paperwork, eyeglasses, mobile telephones, wallet, keys, or agenda

☐ Often leaves things behind

☐ Loses papers for work

☐ Loses notes, lists, or telephone numbers

☐ Loses time searching for things

☐ Gets in a panic if people move my things around

☐ Stores things where they don't belong

8. I am often easily distracted.

☐ Difficulty shutting off external stimuli

☐ After I am distracted, it isn't easy to pick up where I left off

☐ Easily distracted by noises or activity

☐ Easily distracted by the conversations of others

☐ Difficulty filtering and/or selecting information I should pay attention to

9. I am often forgetful in daily activities.

☐ Forgets appointments or other obligations

☐ Needs frequent reminders for appointments

☐ Forgets keys, agenda, and other important possessions

☐ Forgets to pay bills or to return calls

☐ Forgets to keep or look at a daily agenda

☐ Forgets to do chores or run errands

☐ Returns home to retrieve forgotten items

☐ Rigid use of lists to ensure things are remembered

Schedule a visit with your physician if you have several checkmarks in four or more areas.

What Adults Need to Know Before and After an ADHD Diagnosis

Deciding to seek a diagnosis for ADHD is fraught with emotions.

Scenario one: You think you have ADHD, but worry you're wrong and fear being told, "You don't have ADHD." You are not alone in this worry. Sadly, it is true, adults are sometimes told they do not have ADHD even when they do because the physicians and psychologists they see for a diagnosis are unfamiliar with how ADHD presents in adults.

Sometimes, an adult was diagnosed with ADHD in childhood but never sought treatment or stopped treatment. When their lives spiral out of control, they finally want treatment for their ADHD. But even with a record of their childhood diagnosis, they may still encounter scenario one.

Scenario two: You think you have ADHD and fear having it confirmed. You would rather have personality quirks than a disorder. The stigma falsely attached to ADHD affects your willingness to be diagnosed. You fear the diagnosis because you do not realize how life-changing, in a good way, diagnosis and treatment will be. With diagnosis and treatment, life gets better.

A psychologist experienced in diagnosing adults with ADHD told me that adults who think they have ADHD are usually correct. However, to ease your mind in advance and provide information to share with your clinician, print out and complete the ADHD-RS (**https://add.org/adhd-questionnaire/**). The maximum score is 54, but the average range for someone with ADHD is between 30-40.

Another good source is the DIVA 5, a structured interview for adult ADHD that is valid and reliable for diagnosing adult ADHD (**https://www.divacenter.eu/DIVA.aspx?id=528**). The website states it is for clinicians trained in its use. Still, I understood it and completed it. It costs about $10 to download and takes 60-90 minutes to complete. Its detail will teach you the manifestations of ADHD, whether the inattentive or hyperactive/impulsive presentation.

Why You Should Believe You Have ADHD Before You Seek a Diagnosis

Reason one: If the physician you see is reluctant to prescribe a *long-acting amphetamine*, the usual treatment for adult ADHD, you can advocate for the correct treatment. Here are the medications and doses your physician should prescribe after diagnosing your ADHD unless he provides a good reason for not doing so.

Drug	Strength
Adderall XR	5 mg, 10 mg, 15 mg, 20mg, 25 mg
Vyvanse	20 mg, 30 mg, 40 mg, 50 mg, 60 mg,

Focalin XR is also an amphetamine, but contains only one amphet-amine salt, dexmethylphenidate, while Adderall and Vyvanse contain four kinds of amphetamine salts.

Typically, you would be started at a low dose and slowly increase it every few days. You can track your improvements by completing the ASRS111 or DIVA5 again and again. A good response would be getting your ASRS score below 18 or a DIVA 5 with fewer check marks. Side effects of the medication should resolve within a month, but if not, you should next try a **long-acting methylphenidate** medication.

Drug	Strength
Concerta	18 mg, 27 mg, 36 mg, 54 mg
Daytrana	10 mg, 15 mg, 20 mg, 30 mg, 40 mg
Ritalin LA	10 mg, 20 mg, 30 mg, 40 mg

From research, we know that stimulants are the most effective treatment for ADHD. It might take several months to find the proper medication or combination of medications at the correct dose for you. There are over 30 medications used to treat ADHD. The two tables list the most popular ones.

Medication dose does not rely on your age, weight, or severity of the condition. What works for one person is not necessarily what works for you. ADHD is very individual in its presentation and treatment. To get a general feel for how people respond to various medications, read reviews at https://www.webmd.com/drugs/2/index. Only after failing with both kinds of stimulant medications should your physician prescribe Strattera or other non-stimulant medications for treating ADHD unless he can explain why he is prescribing something else for you.

Reason two: The longer you went with untreated ADHD, the more likely you are to have co-morbid depression and/or anxiety. If the physician diagnoses depression along with your ADHD, he might want to treat the depression first. About 25% of adults with untreated ADHD have depression. Treatment is more effective if both, not just the depression, get treated together. If you have anxiety, which almost 50% of adults with untreated ADHD report having, treatment of your ADHD may reduce your anxiety. In that case you won't need a different medication for your anxiety. But if you do, the physician should treat your anxiety after seeing how much it resolves with the ADHD medication.

Reason three: The physician will not diagnose your ADHD and has bizarre explanations for why they won't. The most common and incorrect explanation is that you are too smart, you did well in school or you graduated from college. Other times the physician believes you have ADHD but won't prescribe a stimulant because he fears you are drug-seeking.

While some people with undiagnosed ADHD have substance abuse histories, this shouldn't prevent a physician from prescribing stimulant medication. The physician can supervise its use. Even people in a drug treatment program have fewer relapses when their ADHD is treated.

If you encounter either of these responses, know that you have seen a physician not knowledgeable about ADHD. You need to find another physician to diagnose and treat you.

If you are evaluated by a physician who doesn't know the latest research on diagnosing and treating adult ADHD, getting help for your troubled life can be delayed for years. This is why it is crucial to work with a knowledgeable clinician. You might find a psychologist to diagnose your ADHD and a physician to treat it, or a physician who both diagnoses and treats you. In either scenario, you want knowledgeable providers who have evaluated and/or treated many adults with ADHD.

How will you find knowledgeable clinicians? Search online ADHD directories, such as:

- chadd.org/professionaldirectory

- directory.additudemag.com

- add.org/professional-directory

That said, be aware that providers pay for their listings. Do further research by visiting the websites of possible candidates and reading online reviews by former patients. If you can't locate an experienced provider near you, explore providers that diagnose and treat adult ADHD remotely via telemed.

Ask these questions to evaluate telemed sources for ADHD:

- Can you diagnose and treat ADHD in adults?

- Who will make my diagnosis and what is their experience diagnosing and treating adults with ADHD?

- Can you prescribe stimulants or only non-stimulant medications?

- Are you approved to provide service in the state where I reside?

- What insurance companies cover your services?

- What percentage of the charges do they pay?

- Do you bill insurance or am I expected to?

- How much does an evaluation cost?

- What are the costs of follow-up appointments?

When you go for an evaluation, bring someone with you who has known you for a while. People with ADHD typically have poor memories, especially of their childhood.

After Your Diagnosis

First and foremost: stay the course.

Don't give up on finding a medication that helps you. Too many get discouraged and don't persist when the first medication doesn't help. Don't let alternate treatments, which research has shown are not effective, tempt you. Persistence usually pays off as over 80% of people with ADHD are helped by medication. People online often ask others what medicine they take or which didn't help them. Remember, an effective medication and dose for someone else with ADHD may not be the proper medication for you.

Get educated about ADHD from reliable sources, such as the websites of ADHDevidence.org, CHADD, ADDA, the Inattentive ADHD Coalition, and ADDitude magazine. Read recommended books, watch videos by Russell Barkley, Ph.D., and Jessica McCabe, and participate in webinars featuring noted ADHD providers and researchers.

Focus on creating good habits: eight hours of sleep each night, one hour of exercise at least three times a week, nutritious meals in moderate amounts, along with mindfulness training to reduce your stress.

Seek support and guidance from others with ADHD. There are several ADHD groups on Facebook and Reddit where people share their experiences.

Consider adding individual coaching or cognitive behavioral therapy to the mix if you struggle to implement new behaviors, continue feeling overwhelmed, or aren't making progress. The websites of the ADHD Coaches Association has a directory of coaches while Psychology Today lists therapists. Most coaches work via zoom, and many therapists do as well.

Related Problems to Watch For

Dr. Oren Mason, a family physician who specializes in treating ADHD and related disorders advises physicians to screen for ADHD when a patient presents with any of the following problems.

If you have issues in any of these areas, you might want to discuss a possible ADHD diagnosis with your family physician:

Clinical

- Depression, bipolar
- Anxiety
- Obsessive compulsive disorder

- Post-traumatic stress disorder
- Poor response to medication for depression
- Alcoholism or alcohol abuse
- Substance abuse
- Nicotine addiction
- Multiple serious injuries
- Two or more sexually transmitted diseases
- Crisis pregnancy
- Medical non-compliance

Social

- Pattern of unstable relationships
- Few friends
- Poor social support network
- School disciplinary problems
- Divorce
- Marital discord
- Unresolved marital issues
- Job loss and underemployment
- Frequent job change
- Arrest or incarceration

Self-Management

- Late for appointments
- Educational under-performance or curtailment
- Multiple moving vehicle accidents
- Impulsive shopping
- Burdensome debts
- Credit overextension
- Financial mismanagement

Note: The information in this article is not intended to be medical advice.

Resources for Readers

ADDitude Magazine
additudemag.com

Attention Deficit Disorder Association
add.org

Adult ADHD Self-Report Screener
add.org/adhd-test/

Russell Barkley, Ph.D. (retired)
Recommended video: *The Importance of Emotion in ADHD*
youtube.com/watch?v=hzhL-FA2vl0

Children and Adults with Attention Deficit Disorder
chadd.org

William Dodson, M.D.
additudemag.com/author/william-dodson-m-d

Stephen Faraone, Ph.D.
ADHDEvidence.org

Edward Hallowell, M.D.
drhallowell.com

Inattentive ADHD Coalition
iadhd.org

Rakesh Jain, M.D., M.P.H.
team-adhd.com

Brendan Mahan, M. Ed., M.S.
ADHDessentials.com

Oren Mason, MD
attentionMD.com

Terry Matlen, ACSW
addconsults.com

Caroline McGuire, M.Ed.
carolinemaguireauthor.com

Thomas Phelan, Ph.D.
123magic.com

John Ratey, M.D.
johnratey.com

About the Author

Cynthia Hammer was born and raised in the factory town of Leominster, Massachusetts. She earned an undergraduate degree in economics at Wheaton College and an MSW from the University of Washington in Seattle, where she focused on geriatric social work.

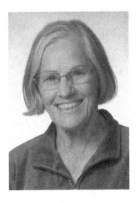

Cynthia's life was significantly affected by inattentive ADHD for many years until she was finally diagnosed at age 49. In 1994 she founded the non-profit organization ADD Resources, which she led for 15 years before retiring.

In 2021, she founded the non-profit, Inattentive ADHD Coalition (www.iadhd.org), because of her concern that too many children and adults with inattentive ADHD remain undiagnosed or incorrectly diagnosed.

She and her husband Steve, the parents of three adult sons, live in Tacoma, Washington, where they enjoy hiking and biking.